MW01049479

MAN'S SUPREME INHERITANCE

F. MATTHIAS ALEXANDER

Published by Left of Brain Books

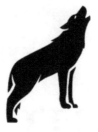

Copyright © 2021 Left of Brain Books

ISBN 978-1-396-32098-9

First Edition

All rights reserved. No part of this publication may be reproduced, distributed, or transmitted in any form or by any means, including photocopying, recording, or other electronic or mechanical methods, without the prior written permission of the publisher, except in the case of brief quotations embodied in critical reviews and certain other noncommercial uses permitted by copyright law. Left of Brain Books is a division of Left of Brain Onboarding Pty Ltd.

Table of Contents

INTRODUCTION

AMONG my intimates I once numbered a boatman, known as Old Sol, or, to his familiars, Sol, simply, without the courtesy title, for he was not notably old. I could not say whether his name was an abbreviated form of Solomon, nor if it were, whether the longer name was baptismal or conferred in later years as a tribute to his undoubted wisdom. I have thought it possible that the name was not an abbreviation at all, but was descriptive of my friend's habit of, optimism in regard to the weather. For to the cockney oarsman who doubtfully contemplated the meteorological conditions on the upper Thames Sol was unwavering in his encouragement. His certainty that the weather would clear and the sun come out was so inspiring that the pale-faced Londoner cheerfully faced the most unpromising outlook, and started out on his uncertain course up-stream buoyed with a beautiful confidence in old Sol's infallibility. But for me and for his other intimates, regular clients whose custom was not dependent on the chances of a fine week-end, Sol had another method. In answer to the usual question, 'Well, Sol, what's it going to do?' he would first look up into the sky, and then step to the edge of the landing-stage and study so much of the horizon as was within his limit of vision; after this careful survey he would deliver his opinion, judicially, and I rarely found him at fault in his prophecy.

Facing my critics, lay and professional, I wish at the outset to disclaim the methods by which Sol invigorated the casual amateur. I am not prophesying unlimited sunshine for every one, without regard to conditions. In this brochure will be found no mention of royal roads, panaceas, or grand specifics. Rather I have attempted to treat every reader as Sol treated his intimates. I have looked into the sky and made a careful survey of the horizon. It is true that I have seen an ideal and the promise of its fulfilment, but my deductions have been drawn with patient care from signs which I have studied with diligence; if I am an optimist, it is because I see the promise of fair weather, and not because I wish to delude the unwary. And with this I will lay down my metaphor and come to a practical statement.

1

I know that I shall be regarded in many quarters as a revolutionary and a heretic, for my theory and practice, though founded on a principle as old as the life of man, are not in accord with, nor even a development of, the tradition which still obtains. But in thus rejecting tradition I am, happily, sustained by something more than an unproved theory. Moreover, on this firm ground I do not stand alone. Though my theory may appear revolutionary and heretical, it is shared by men of attainment in science and medicine. On a small scale I have made many converts, and in now making appeal to a wider circle I am upheld by the knowledge that what I have to say can no longer be classed as an isolated opinion.

Not that I should have hesitated to come forward now, even if I had been without support. During the past six years I have built up a practice in London which has reached the bounds of my capacity. This work has not been done by any advancement of a wavering hypothesis. I have had cases brought to me as the result of the failure of many kinds of treatment, of rest cures, relaxation cures, hypnotism, faith cures, physical culture, and the ordinary medical prescriptions—and in the treatment of these cases, in my own observations, and in the appreciation of the patients themselves, I have had abundant opportunity to prove to my own satisfaction that in its application to present needs my theory has stood the test of practice in every circumstance and condition.

That the limits imposed by the present work render it woefully inadequate I am quite willing to admit, but the necessity for a certain urgency has been forced upon me, and I have deemed it wiser to outline my subject at once rather than wait for the time when I shall be ready to publish my larger work, and I have at the same time reprinted in this brochure two earlier pamphlets, namely one on Respiratory Re-Education and one on the Kinæsthetic Systems.

With regard to the larger work I can say little here, save that it will be the natural continuation of this brochure which may well serve as a preface. I have, now, space sufficient only to indicate the foundations of my belief, but I hope very soon to present the superstructure complete in every detail. In this brochure I have confined myself to the primary argument and indicated the direction in which we may find physical completeness. In the work which will follow I will deal with the detailed evidence of the application of my theory to life, of cases and cures, and all the substance of experience.

There are, however, many reasons why I should hesitate no longer in making my preliminary appeal, and chief among them is the appalling physical deterioration that can be seen by any intelligent observer who will walk the streets of London, for example, and note the form and aspect of the average individuals who make up the crowd. So much for the surface. What inferences can we not draw from the statistics? What are we to make of the disproportionate increase of insanity, cancer, and appendicitis, which appears undeniable, to take these three instances only? For the increase progresses despite the fact that we have taken the subject seriously to heart. Now I would not fall into the common fallacy of *post hoc ergo propter hoc*, and say that because the increase of these evils has gone hand-in-hand with our endeavours to raise the standard by physical-culture theories, relaxation exercises, rest cures, and *hoc genus omne*, therefore the one is the result of the other; but I do maintain—lacking more definite proof on the first point—that if physical culture exercises, etc., had done all that they were hoped to do, they must be considered a complete failure in the checking of the three evils I have instanced.

Are these troubles still to increase, then? Are we to wait while the bacteriologist patiently investigates the nature of these diseases, till he triumphantly isolates some characteristic germ and announces that here, at last, is the dread bacillus of cancer? Should we even then be any nearer a cure? Could we rely on inoculation, and if we could, in this case, what is to be the end? Are we to be inoculated against every known disease till our bodies become depressed and enervated sterilities, incapable of action on their own account? I pray not, for such a physical condition would imply a mental condition even more pitiable. The science of bacteriology has its uses, but they are the uses of research rather than of application. Bacteriology reveals the agents active in disease, but it says nothing about the conditions which permit these agents to become active. Therefore I look to that wonderful instrument, the human body, for the true solution of our difficulty, an instrument so inimitably adaptable, so full of marvellous potentialities of resistance and recuperation that it is able, when properly used, to overcome all the forces of disease.

In this thing I do not address myself to any one class or section of the community. I have tried in what follows to avoid, so far as may be, any terminology, any medical or scientific phrases and technicalities, and to speak to the entire intelligent public. I wish the scheme I have here adumbrated to be taken up universally, and not to be restricted to the advantage of any body, medical or otherwise. I wish to do away with such teachers as I am myself. My place in the present economy is due to a misunderstanding of the causes of our present physical disability, and when this disability is finally eliminated, the specialized practitioner will have no place, no uses. This may be a dream of the future, but in its beginnings it is now capable of realization. Every man, woman and child holds the possibility of physical perfection; it rests with each of us to attain it by personal understanding and effort.

F. MATTHIAS ALEXANDER

22 ARMY AND NAVY MANSIONS,
VICTORIA STREET, S.W.

I.
FROM PRIMITIVE CONDITIONS
TO PRESENT NEEDS

'Our contemporaries of this and the rising generation appear to be hardly aware that we are witnessing the last act of a long drama, a tragedy and a comedy in one, which is being silently played, with no fanfare or trumpets or roll of drums, before our eyes on the stage of history. Whatever becomes of the savages, the curtain must descend on savagery for ever.' — J. G. FRAZER

THE long process of evolution still moves quietly to its unknown accomplishment; struggle and starvation, the hard fight for existence working with fine impartiality, remorselessly eliminates the weak and defective; new variations are developed and old types no further adaptable become extinct and thus life fighting for life improves towards a sublimation we cannot foresee. But at some period of the world's history an offshoot of a dominant type began to develop new powers that were destined to change the face of the world. What first influenced the trend of that new development we can only guess, dimly. It may have been as a modern French writer[1] suggests, that courage was a determining factor, a suggestion that is at once consistent with our surmises as to the prevailing conditions and acceptable to our intellectual pride. Whatever the influence which first begot these new powers, they held strange potentialities, and, among others, that which now immediately concerns us—the potentiality to counteract the force of evolution itself.

This is, indeed, at once the greatest triumph of our intellectual growth and the self-constituted danger which threatens us from within. Man has arisen above nature, bent circumstance to his will, and striven in antagonism to the mighty force of evolution. He has pried into the great workshop interfered with the machinery, endeavouring to become master of its action and to

---

[1] *Notre Père des Bois, La Forêt Nuptiale, La Caverne*, par Ray Nyst. (Paris, 1900, etc.)

control the workings of its component parts. But the machine has as yet proved too intricate for his complete comprehension, slowly he has learned the uses of a few parts which he is able to operate, but it is only a small fraction of the whole.

What then is man's position to-day, and what is his danger? His position is this: By emerging from the contest with nature he has ceased to be a natural animal. He has evolved curious powers of discrimination, of choice, and of construction. He has changed his environment, his food, and his whole manner of living. He has inquired into the laws which govern heredity and into the causes of disease. But still his knowledge is limited, and his emergence incomplete. The power of the force we know as evolution still holds him in chains, though man has loosened his bonds and may at last free himself entirely. Thus we come to man's danger.

Evolution—a term we use here and elsewhere in this connection as that which is best understood to indicate the whole operation of natural selection and all that it connotes—has two clearly defined functions: by the one of these it develops; by the other destroys. By an infinitely slow action it has developed such wonders as the human eye or hand; by a process somewhat less tedious it allows any organ that has become useless to perish, such as the pineal eye or (in process) the vermiform appendix, and if we can estimate the future course, the teeth and hair.

By the change he has effected in his mode of life, man is no longer necessarily dependent upon his physical organism for the means of his subsistence, and in cases where he is still so dependent, such as those of the agriculturist, the artisan, and others who earn a living by manual labour, he employs his muscles in new ways, in mechanical repetitions of the same act, or in modes of labour which are far removed from those called forth by primitive conditions. In some ways the physical type which represents the rural labouring population is, in my opinion, even more degenerate than the type we find in cities, and mentally there can be no comparison between the two. The truth is that man, whether living in town or country, has changed his habitat and with it his habits, and in so doing has put himself in a new danger, for though evolution may be cruel in its methods, it is the cruelty of a discipline without which our bodies become relaxed, our muscles atrophied, and our functions put out of gear.

The antagonism of conscious as opposed to natural selection[2] has now been in existence for many thousands of years, but it is only within the last century or less that the effect upon man's constitution has become so marked that this danger of deterioration or decay has been thrust upon the attention, not only of scientific observers, but of the average, intelligent individual. No examination of history is necessary in this place to set out a reason for this comparatively sudden realisation of physical unfitness. Briefly, the civilization of the past hundred years has been unlike the many that have preceded it in that it has not been confined to any single nation or empire. In the past history of the world an intellectual civilization such as that of Egypt, Persia, Greece, or Rome, perished from internal causes, and chief among them was a moral and physical deterioration which rendered the nation unequal to a struggle with younger, more vigorous and—this is important—wilder, more natural peoples. Thus we have good cause for believing that the danger we have indicated, though still incipient only, was a determining cause in the downfall of past civilizations. But we must not overlook the fact that destructive wars and devastating plagues held sway in the earlier history of mankind, and while the latter acted as an instrument of evolution in destroying the unfit, the former by decreasing the population threw a burden of initiative and energy on the remnant, necessitating the use of active, physical qualities in the business of all kinds of production.

Now the conditions have altered. Greater scientific attainments in every direction than have ever been known, have combated, and will probably in the future overcome the devastating diseases which have decimated the populations of cities; while a higher ethical ideal tends ever to oppose the horrible and repugnant barbarism of war which, as civilization grows, constantly spreading, even to the peoples of the Orient, becomes to our senses more and more fratricidal, a fight of brother against brother.

---

[2] It should, however, be clearly understood in this connection that certain laws of natural selection must, so far as we can see, always hold good; and it would not be advisable to alter them even if it were possible. For example, that curious law may be cited which ordains the attraction of opposites in mating and so maintains nature's average. The attraction which a certain type of woman has for a certain type of man, and *vice versa*, is, in my opinion, a fundamental law, and any attempt to regulate it would be harmful to the race. This, however, is no argument against the regulation or prevention of marriages between the physically and mentally unfit.

A hundred years ago, Malthus, a prophet, if not a seer, recognised our danger, and within the past quarter of a century a dozen theorists have proposed remedies less stringent than those proposed by Malthus, but almost equally futile. Among the theorists are those reactionaries (consciously or unconsciously) who advocate the simple life by a return to natural food and conditions, in endlessly various suggestions. To them in their search for natural foods and conditions we would point out that countless generations separate us from primitive man, a lapse of time during which our functions have become gradually adapted to new habits and environment; and that if it were possible by universal agreement for the peoples of Europe to return instantly to primitive methods of living, the effect would be no less disastrous than the reversal of the process, the sudden thrusting of our civilization upon savage tribes whereby—to quote one or two recent examples only—the aborigines of North America, New Zealand, and Japan (the Ainu tribes) have become, or are rapidly becoming, extinct.

When we point out man's power of adaptability in this connection, therefore, the emphasis is thrown on the slowness with which that adaptability is passed on to our descendants and the relative permanence of the new powers acquired. For our purpose the argument remains good whether we admit or deny the inheritability of acquired characteristics, our point being that in either case the process is necessarily a slow one, though it is plainly more rapid if the hypothesis be true.[3]

It becomes necessary, if we would be consistent, to reject at once all propositions for improving our future well-being, which can by any possibility be described as reactionary. Even in this brief résumé of man's history one tendency stands out clearly enough, the tendency to advance. When that first offshoot from a dominant type began to develop new powers of intellect a form was initiated which must either progress or perish. Atavism must be counteracted by the powers of the mind, and reaction is a form of atavism. No return to earlier conditions can increase our knowledge of the secret springs of life, can aid our formulation of world-laws by the understanding of which we may hope to control the future course of development.

---

[3] For a further statement of one aspect of heredity see chapter vi. of this brochure.

In the mind of man lies the secret of his ability to resist, to conquer and finally to govern the circumstance of his life, and only by the discovery of that secret will he ever be able to realize completely the perfect condition of *mens sana in corpore sano*.

II.
PRIMITIVE REMEDIES AND THEIR DEFECTS

'... Having heard that Henry Taylor was ill, Carlyle rushed off from London to Sheen with a bottle of medicine, which had done Mrs. Carlyle good, without in the least knowing what was ailing Henry Taylor, or for what the medicine was useful.' — *Life of Tennyson*.

THE danger of mental, nervous, and muscular debility, the outcome of the conditions which obtain as the result of the trend of our development, has been widely recognized during the past fifty years; and we must turn aside for a moment to consider certain phases of its treatment as indicated by the well-known and widely applied terms 'physical culture,' 'relaxation,' and 'deep-breathing.'

With regard to 'physical culture,' it must be clearly understood that I do not allude to any one system of practice, but speak in the widest terms, terms which are applicable alike to the most primitive forms of dumb-bell exercise, or to the most elaborate series of evolutions designed to counteract the effect of a particular malady. (But lest my application of the term be misunderstood, I will define that 'physical-culture,' where so written and between inverted commas, stands for 'a series of *mechanical* exercises, simple or complicated, designed to strengthen a bodily function by the development of a set of muscles or of the complete system of muscles'; but when I use the words physical culture, currently and without a hyphen, I denote a general system for the improvement of the entire physical economy, by a just co-ordination and control of all the parts of the system, particularly excluding any method which tends to the hypertrophy of any one energy without regard to the balance of the whole).

In the first place it will be recognized from what I have already said that the whole theory upon which the present 'physical culture' school is based is but another aspect of the reversion to nature which we have stigmatized as a form of atavism. It is an attempt to stiffen the new garment of our intellectual development by lining it with the old fabric of so-called nature exercise. 'Physical-culture,' as defined, is what one might term the obvious, uninspired method which naturally presents itself as a remedy for the ills arising from an artificial condition. The logic of it is of the simplest, and arises from the major premise that bodily defects arise from the disuse and misuse of muscles and energies in an artificial civilization, which muscles and energies in a natural state are continually being called upon to provide the means of livelihood.

From this it seems obvious to argue that if we contrive an artificial mechanical means of exercising these muscles for, say, one, two, or three hours a day, they will resume their natural functions, and so.... The lacuna cannot be satisfactorily filled. If we carry on the argument to its logical conclusion the fallacy is made evident. For the method arising from this argument creates civil war within the body. There is no co-ordination, and the outcome must be strife; but the point will be made clearer by an instance which must be taken to represent a broadly typical case, an allegory rather than a special example of particular application.

Let us take the case of, say, John Doe, whose work keeps him indoors from nine A.M. to six P.M., and makes a very urgent call upon his mental and nervous powers. By the time he is thirty-five, possibly five or ten years sooner, John Doe is suffering from anæmia, indigestion, nervous debility, lassitude, insomnia, heart weakness, and heaven only knows what other troubles. His bodily functions are irregular, his muscular system partly atrophied and unresponsive, his nerves irritated, and, there is really no better word, 'jumpy.'

Incidentally I must note, also, that his mind is inoperative in many directions. He has a bad mental attitude towards the physical acts of everyday life. For him his body is a mechanism (the intricate workings of which he never pauses to examine) to be driven or forced through a certain series of evolutions similar in kind to those it has always performed within his experience, and when this mechanism fails it is to be forced on again by tonics and stimulants or given a 'rest,' which is followed by a return to the old methods of propulsion.

However, John Doe, who has postponed seeking a remedy already far too long, at last takes a course of 'physical-culture,' but his time is severely limited, and his exercises are confined to an hour or two morning and evening. At first he may say that he feels a wonderful benefit and probably advises every friend he meets in the city to follow his example. I am quite willing to grant that Doe may be benefited, I will even admit that if he continues his exercises, it is possible he may not fall back into the same state of nervous prostration into which he fell originally; but what I wish to make quite clear is that his cure did not in itself possess the elements of permanence, that it was merely a tinkering or botching of the fabric of his body. For if we consider his case from a purely detached standpoint we must see that Doe has attempted to develop two systems or modes of life which were not mutually agreeable. On the one hand, for two, three, or four hours a day, he was occupied in mechanically developing his muscular system without making any difference in the manner in which he drove his machine, and stimulating and accelerating the supply of blood which therefore required increased oxygenation or reinforced lung power; he was, in brief, exercising those functions and energies which in a primitive state would have been called upon during the greater part of his waking life to supply him with food. On the other hand, for the remaining twelve hours or so during which he was engaged in the business of his profession, in the eating of meals and in reading, playing indoor games, or in similar sedentary occupations, the newly developed powers were being neglected, and a call was made upon the old nervous energies and centres of control. John Doe's physical body thus had two existences—excluding the natural condition of sleep—one fiercely active, muscular, dynamic; the other sedentary, nervous, static.

These two existences are not correlated, they are antagonistic, they do not mutually support each other, they conflict. John Doe's body becomes the scene of a civil war, and the heart, lungs, and other semi-automatic organs are in a state of perpetual readjustment to opposing conditions, as they are called upon to support one side or the other in the perpetual combat. Such a condition cannot tend in the long run to the improvement of mankind as a whole.

For, as I shall show later,[4] in the case of John Doe, and in all parallel cases, the consciousness of the person concerned is not changed in regard to the use of the muscular mechanism. Let him exercise even for six hours daily, yet immediately on taking up his ordinary occupations once more, he will revert to the same muscular habits he has already acquired in connection with such occupations. It is not difficult to see that John Doe has a wrong mental

---

[4] For a fuller analysis of this see p. *33 et seq.* of this brochure.

attitude, towards the uses of his muscular mechanism in the acts of everyday life. He has been using muscles to do work for which they were never intended, while others, which should have been continuously employed, remain undeveloped, inert, imperfectly controlled. He is, in truth, suffering from mental and physical delusions with regard to the uses of his body. To quote but one of a dozen instances of his lack of recognition of the true uses and functions of his muscular system, we shall notice that when he thrusts his head forward or throws it back, his shoulders always accompany the movement in either direction, this movement of the shoulders being entirely unconscious, and made without any recognition of the fact that they are being moved. Now, in this condition of mental and physical delusion, the unfortunate man tries to do something with these mechanisms which he is unable to control, in the hope that by merely performing certain physical exercises, he can restore his body to a condition of perfect physical health.

Some perception of the evils we have thus briefly summarized has been awakened in the minds of the more earnest thinkers during the last few years, and as a result the systems of exercises display a clearly marked tendency towards modification, they have lessened their muscle-tensing violence, and have become, and are becoming, ever less and less strenuous physical acts. Thus we find 'physical-culture' advocates who a few years ago insisted upon the use of dumb-bells—in some cases dumb-bells increasing in weight over a graduated series of exercises—now emphasize the necessity for *gentle* exercises, and the dumb-bell is not mentioned, which is, perhaps, as good a proof as any of the truth of my contentions.

My next instance, namely, 'relaxation,' is even less efficient. The usual procedure is to instruct the pupil (who is either sitting or lying on the floor) to relax, or to do what he (or she) understands by relaxing. The result is invariably collapse. For relaxation really means a due tension of the parts of the muscular system intended by nature to be constantly more or less tensed, together with a relaxation of those parts intended by nature to be more or less relaxed, a condition which is readily secured in practice by adopting what I have called in my other writings, the position of mechanical advantage.[5] But, apart from an incorrect understanding of the proper condition natural to the

---

[5] See 'Re-education of the Kinæsthetic Systems' incorporated in this volume, p. *43 et seq.*

various muscles, the theory of relaxation, like that of the rest cure, makes a wrong assumption, and if either system is persisted in, there must inevitably follow a general lowering of vitality, which will be felt the moment regular duties are taken up again, and which will soon bring about the return of the old troubles in an exaggerated form.

The last remedy mentioned at the opening of this chapter was 'deep-breathing.' This is a later form of 'physical-culture' development, and is, in effect, a modification in the right direction. It is the consistent outcome of the perception that strenuous, forcing, muscular exercises were resulting in new and possibly greater evils than those they professed to cure. 'Deep-breathing' is indeed a step in the right direction, but only a step, because, while it does not always do serious harm, and in some instances, perhaps, a certain amount of good, it does not go to the root of the matter, the eradication of defects; nor take cognisance of the most important factor in the scheme of physical co-ordination. What the radical factor is I shall deal with in detail in my next chapter, but I will first glance briefly over the chief phases of the argument so far as it has been unfolded.

In imagination we have seen man through the darkness which covers his first appearance on the earth, the early Miocene man. As we have figured him he was a creature of simple needs, and of a vigorous bodily habit, an animal in all save that spark of self-consciousness which burned feebly in his primitive, but increasing and differentiating brain. Again we have a somewhat clearer vision of him with wider powers of courage and cunning, adapting weapons to his use, and so specializing the functions of his mind through a long two million years, through palæolithic and neolithic periods into the age of bronze where he has become a reasoning, designing creature, with powers of imagination and idealization which are still turned, however, to physical uses.

And, at last, we reach the differentiation of man from man and class from class which marks the historical period of civilization, the period of dwelling in cities, the adaptability to new and specialized habits, of labour that makes little or no call upon the physical capacities, of food procured without energy; the period when the slow process of evolution, which has resulted in the product of a new and marvellous instrument of self-conscious, directive powers, was becoming gradually superseded by that which it had brought forth.

III.
SUB-CONSCIOUSNESS AND INHIBITION

'You can have neither a greater nor a less dominion over yourself.' —
LEONARDO DA VINCI.

WITHIN thirty years we have evolved a new science, the science of psychology. A generation since psychology was subject-matter only for the philosopher, the metaphysician, the poet, or the ecclesiastic, now it is being investigated in the laboratory by tests of sensibility, reaction times and other responses to stimulation too technical to be explained here; tests carried out by means of elaborate and intricate instruments and machinery designed to weigh *the hidden springs of life* in the balance. The phrase I have italicized is purposely vague, for I have no wish to fall foul of a terminology, nor to make any *a priori* assumption which might involve me in controversial matters completely outside my province. At the same time, I see clearly that some convenient phrase will become necessary, and I will therefore adopt one which is at least familiar and within certain limits descriptive enough, namely the 'sub-conscious self.'

It may seem strange that one should look to any formally organized science, such as psychology now is to a science working in a laboratory with mechanical appliances, for any elucidation of a question which has for so long been regarded as strictly within the domain of the priest. But science, as Tyndal said, is only another name for common-sense, and a little consideration will show that the postulate I have insisted upon, namely, the growth and progress of intellectual control, demands that this admirable quality of common-sense, or reason, should be applied to the elucidation of this all-important problem. Unhappily, psychology, from which we hope so much, is yet in its infancy, and therefore, though I would be guided as far as possible by its methods, I must transcend its present limits in the consideration of the sub-conscious self.

15

The concepts which have grown up round this designation are, in many cases, curiously concrete in form. Much error has sprung from that earnest and well-intentioned work of the late F.W.H. Myers, *Human Personality and its Survival after Bodily Death*. Mr. Myers figured an entity within an entity; and his work, though inductive in form, was *a priori* in method, for he had conceived the picture of a subjective personality taking shape within an objective, material shell, and controlled his evidence to a definite, preconceived end.

The fallacies of Myers have been exposed again and again; his argument is intrinsically unsound, and when put to the test of newer knowledge his hypothesis fails to explain the fact. But because Myers' conception was so graphic and credible it took a strong hold upon the popular imagination, a hold, which the eight years following the publication of *Human Personality* has not weakened in the minds of a great number of people, full though these years have been of discovery and new knowledge. It is for this reason that I have reverted to Myers' conception of the sub-conscious, or, as he called it, 'sub-liminal self,' inasmuch as I wish it to be clearly understood from the outset that I use the designation to denote an entirely different concept. Indeed, anyone who has followed my argument to this point must have inferred the trend of my purpose, namely, that as the intellectual powers of man extend, we progress in the direction of *conscious control*. The gradual control of evolution by the child of its production, has pointed always to this end, and by this means, and by this alone, can the human race continue in the full enjoyment of its physical powers and forfeit no fraction of its progressive intellectual ideal.

It will inevitably be asked at this stage what I intend when I speak of that which I have consented to designate the 'sub-conscious self,' and I must therefore answer that question to the best of my ability, even though I have to leave for a moment the limits of proved fact and tread on the wider ground of hypothesis. I do not purpose, however, to overburden my theory with the detail of evidence, and what follows must therefore be taken as an inclusive statement, much of which I could prove conclusively in a larger work, while the unproved remnant must necessarily await confirmation from the researches of future investigators in the domains of psychology. Briefly then we must see that the sub-conscious self is not a possession peculiar to man, but that it is in fact more active, in many ways more finely developed in the animal world. In some animals the consciousness of danger is so keen that we have attributed it to prescience. The fear of fire (in the prairies), of flood, or of the advance of some natural danger threatening the existence of the animal, is evidenced far ahead of any signs perceptible by human senses, and since we cannot (except sentimentally) attribute powers of conscious reasoning to the animal world, it is evident that this 'fore-knowledge' is due to a delicate co-ordination of animal senses. Again we see that animals which have not had their powers dulled by many generations of domestication make the majority of their movements, as we say, 'instinctively.' They can judge the length of a leap with astonishing accuracy, or take the one certain chance of escape among the many apparent possibilities open to them without an instant's hesitation; and these powers are evidenced in many cases within a few hours or minutes after the birth of the animal; they are admittedly not the outcome of experience.

The whole argument for the evidence of the possession of a sub-conscious self by animals can be elaborated to any length, and depends upon facts of observation made over a long period of time. The few examples I have here cited merely illustrate that side of the question which throws into prominence the point of what we may call abnormal powers, or powers which seem to transcend those of human reason so far as it has been developed. It is this appearance of transcendent qualities in the human sub-consciousness which misled Myers, who did not pause to apply his allegory of the sub-conscious entity to the animal world, an application which would have tended to prove that the 'soul' (for that is what Myers really intended, however carefully he may have avoided the actual word) of the animal was more highly developed than that of man.

I may, however, assume that the point has been already sufficiently demonstrated, for I am eager to come to the point which marks the differentiation of man from the animal world, and which is first clearly evidenced in the use of the reasoning, intellectual powers of inhibition.

Now it is evident that in the earlier stages of man's development, the inhibition of the sub-conscious animal powers was frequently a source of danger and of death. Reason not yet sufficiently instructed and far-seeing was an inefficient pilot, and sometimes laid the ship aback when she would have

17

kept before the wind if left to herself. To abandon the metaphor, the control was imperfect, wavered between two alternatives and rejecting the guidance of instinct, suffered, it may be, destruction. But the necessity for conscious control grew as the conditions of life departed ever more and more from those of the wild state. This, plainly, for many reasons, but chief of all by reason of the limitations enforced by the social habit which grew out of the need for co-operation.

This point must be briefly elaborated, for it outlines the birth of inhibition in its application to everyday life; and in so doing demonstrates the growth of the principle of conscious control which, after countless thousands of years, we are but now beginning to appreciate and understand.

It is true that we have evidence of conscious inhibition in a pure state of nature. The wild cat stalking its quarry inhibits the desire to spring prematurely, and controls to a deliberate end its eagerness for instant gratification of a natural appetite. But in this, and in the many other similar instances such instinctive acts of inhibition have been developed through long ages of necessity. The domestic kitten of a few weeks old, which has never been dependent on its own efforts for a single meal, will exhibit the same instinct. In animals the inherited power is there; in man also the power is there as a matter of physical inheritance, but with what added possibilities as the accumulated product of experience from the conscious use of this wonderful force.

The first experience must have come to man very early in his development. So soon as any act was proscribed and punishment meted out for its performance, or so soon as a reward was consciously sought though its attainment necessitated realized, personal danger—there must have been a deliberate, conscious inhibition of natural desires, which further enforced a similar restraint of muscular, physical functioning. As the needs of society widened, this necessity for the daily, hourly inhibition of natural desires increased to a bewildering extent on the prohibitive side. There grew up first 'taboos,' and then the rough formulation of moral and social law, and on the other side an ambition for larger powers which encouraged qualities of emulation and ambition.

Among the infinite diversity of these influences, natural appetites, and the modes of gratifying them, were ever more and more held in subjection, and the sub-conscious self or instinct which initiated every action in the lower animal world fell under the subjection of the conscious, dominating intellect or will, and in the process we must not overlook one fact of supreme importance: man still progressed physically and mentally. This control acquired by the conscious mind broke no great law of nature, known or unknown; for if this acquired control had been in conflict with any of those great and, to us, as yet, incomprehensible forces which have ruled the evolution of species, the animal we call man would have become extinct as did those early saurian types which failed to fulfil the purpose of development and perished before man's first appearance on this earth.

But any exact definition of the sub-conscious self necessitates a clearer comprehension of the terms 'will,' 'mind,' and 'matter,' which may or may not be different aspects of one and the same force. More than two thousand years of philosophy have left the metaphysician still vaguely speculating as to the relations of these three essentials, and, personally, I am not very hopeful of any solution from this source. The investigation, though still in its infancy in this form, has taken the shape of an exact science, and it is to that science of psychology as now understood, that I look to the elucidation of many difficult problems in the future. Without touching on the uncertain ground of speculative philosophy, I will try, however, to be as definite as may be with regard to my conception of the sub-conscious self.

In the first place, great prominence has been given to the conception of the sub-conscious self as an entity within an entity by the argument as to its absolute control of the bodily functions. In support of this argument all the evidence of hypnotism and the various forms of auto-suggestion and faith-healing has been advanced. Under the first heading we have been told that under the direction of the hypnotist the ordinary functions of the body may be controlled or superseded, as for instance, that a wound may be formed and bleed without mechanically breaking the skin, or that a wound may be healed more rapidly than is consistent with the ordinary course of nature as exemplified in the body of the subject.[6] Under the second heading, which

---

[6] Cf. *Hypnotism*, by Albert Moll. Good cases of suppuration, blistering, and bleeding, as the result of suggestion without any preliminary abrasion of the skin, are those supplied by the records of Professor Forel's experiments at the Zurich Lunatic Asylum These experiments

includes all forms of self-suggestion, we have had examples of what is known as stigmatization,[7] or the appearance on the body of hysterical and obsessed subjects of some imitation of the five sacred wounds; and the instances of cures which seem to our uninstructed minds as miraculous, due by inference to the power of faith, are so numerous that no special example need be cited.

These and many kindred phenomena have been explained on the hypothesis that the hidden entity when commanded by the will is able to exert an all-powerful influence either beneficent or malignant; the obscure means by which the command may be enforced being variously described. We see, at once, that the conception of a hidden entity is the primitive explanation which first occurs to the puzzled mind.

We find the same tendency in the many curious superstitions of the savage who endows every bird, beast, stone and tree with powers of evil or of good, and discovers a 'hidden entity,' all of a piece with this conception of the sub-conscious self, in a piece of wood that he has cut from a tree, or a lump of clay that he had modelled into the rude shape of man, bird, or beast.

My own conception is rather of the unity than the diversity of life. And since any attempt to define the term Life would be presumptuous, the definition being beyond the scope of man's present ability, I will merely say that life in this connection must be read in the widest application conceivable. And it appears to me that all we know of the evolution or development of life goes to show that it has progressed, and will continue to progress in the direction of self-consciousness.[8] If we grant the unity of life and the tendency of its evolution, it follows that all the manifestation of what we have called the 'sub-conscious self' are functions of the vital essence or life-force, which functions are passing from automatic or conscious to reasoning or conscious control. (This conception does not necessarily imply any distinction between the thing controlled and the control itself. This may be inferred from the use

---

were conducted on the person of a nurse who is described as the daughter of healthy country people, and not a hysterical subject.

[7] There is much evidence on this point, some of it conflicting, but the main fact must be considered above question.

[8] Cf. Herbert Spencer, *Education*, chapter xi, 'Humanity has progressed solely by self-instruction'

of the word 'self-conscious,' but the further elucidation of this side of the theory is not germane to the present argument.)

Now I am quite prepared to accept phenomena of the kind I have instanced, such as unusual cures effected by hypnotism, and by the somewhat allied methods of the various forms of faith-healing; but I do deny, and most emphatically deny, that either procedure is in any way necessary to produce the same, or even more unusual, phenomena.[9] In other words, I say that man may in time obtain complete conscious control of every function of the body without—as is implied by the word 'conscious'—going into any trance induced by hypnotic means, and without any paraphernalia of making reiterated assertions or statements of belief.

Apart from my practical experience of the harm that so often results from hypnotic and suggestive treatment, an experience sufficient to demonstrate the dangers of applying these methods to a large majority of cases, I found my objection to these practices on a broad and, I believe, incontrovertible basis. This is that the obtaining of trance is a prostitution and degradation of the objective mind; that it ignores and debases the chief curative agent, the apprehension of the patient's conscious mind; and that it is in direct contradiction to the governing principle of evolution, the great law of self-preservation by which the instinct of animals has been trained, as it were, to meet and overcome the imminent dangers of everyday existence. In man this desire for life is an influence in therapeutics, so strong that I can hardly exaggerate its potentiality, and it is, moreover, an influence that can be readily awakened and developed. The will to live has in one experience of mine lifted a woman almost from the grave, a woman who had been operated upon and practically abandoned as dead by her surgeons. A passing thought flashing across a brain that had all but abandoned the struggle for existence, a sudden consciousness that her children might not be well cared for if she died, was sufficient to reawaken the desire for life, and to revivify a body which no medical skill could have saved.[10] But there is no need to quote instances; the

---

[9] Moreover, I deny that hypnotism can possibly succeed except in comparatively rare instances. It is not universal in its applicability.

[10] Two years later this woman came to me in a state of collapse, the result of the after effects of a bad attack of pleurisy. She proved an admirable patient, and is now in perfect

fact is recognized yet how small is the attempt made to make use of and control so potent a force! The same argument may be applied, also, to the prostration of the mind as a factor in the popular rest cures which really seek to put the mind, the great regenerating force, out of action.

Returning to my definition of the sub-conscious self, it will be seen that I regard it as a manifestation of the partly conscious vital essence, functioning at times very vividly, but on the whole incompletely, and from this postulate it follows that our endeavours should be directed to perfecting the self-consciousness of this vital essence. The perfect attainment of this object in every individual would imply a mental and physical ability, and a complete immunity from disease that is still a dream of the future. But once the road is pointed, we must forsake the many bypaths however fascinating, bypaths which lead at last to an impasse, and necessitate a return in our own footsteps. Instead of this we must devote our energies along the indicated road, a road that presents, it is true, many difficulties, and is not straight and easy to traverse, but a road that nevertheless leads to an ideal of mental and physical completeness almost beyond our imaginings.

We look towards the goal, and it is best to seek the highest and be content with no less, but at the same time it is necessary time it is necessary that we should consider the practical detail of our journey. What follows may seem trivial by comparison with the high endeavour I have outlined, but it is the triviality of the

I wish to point the road still more clearly, and to show how every man and woman may learn to walk upon it.

---

health. She was a magnificent instance of a case in which the power was there, finely developed, but not the knowledge which would enable her to make full use of that power.

IV.
CONSCIOUS CONTROL

'The philosophy of the eternal values cannot be anything else but the systematic deduction of all possible absolutely valid values from one principle, and for us this one principle is now founded on the deepest rock of our inner world—on the will to have a world which is self-asserting.' — HUGO MUNSTERBERG, *The Eternal Values*

'Man one harmonious soul of many a soul
Whose nature is its own divine control.' — SHELLEY

ONE of the most recent phases of popular, as opposed to scientific, thought has been that which has endeavoured to teach the control of the mind. Generally this teaching has been spoken of as the 'New Thought' movement, though certain of its precepts may be found in Marcus Aurelius. This movement has had, and is still having, a considerable vogue in America, and the influence of it has been felt in England, many of the writings of its exponents having been published here within the last fifteen or twenty years. The object of the teaching is to promote the habit of 'right thinking,' which is to be obtained by the control of the mind. The 'New Thought' teaches that certain ideas, such as fear, worry, anger, are to be rigidly excluded from the mind and the attention fixed upon their opposites, such as courage, complacency, calm. With certain of the tendencies expressed in this movement I am in sympathy, but following the usual progression of such movements, the 'New Thought' is losing sight of the principle—which was, indeed, never fully grasped—and is becoming involved in a species of dogma, the rigidity of which is, in my opinion, directly opposed to the primary object. One of its earlier and most capable exponents,[11] however, marked the principle with a phrase, and by naming one of his works *In Tune with the Infinite*, gave permanence to the central idea, though more recent writers in

---

[11] Ralph Waldo Trine.

embroidering the theme have lost sight of the original thesis. Moreover, I have not found in the 'New Thought' a proper consideration of cause and effect in treating the mental and physical in combination. There is, and has always been, exhibited the fallacy of considering the mental and physical as in some sense antitheses, which are opposed to each other and make war, whereas the two must be considered, at least, as entirely interdependent, and, in my opinion, even more closely knit than is implied by such a phrase.

I have touched briefly on the movement here because it emphasizes the fact that we are dimly grasping at a truth and paralyzing our attempts to hold it by the premature assumption that we have it safe at last. At the same time I believe that underlying the teachings of these recent movements, 'New Thought' and, generally, 'Faith-healing' (and in these two closely allied influences I include all the offshoots and subdivisions), there is some apprehension of an essential, an apprehension which is liable to lose its grip by reason of the dogma and ritual that has grown up and tends to obscure the one fundamental.

All these sects, parties, societies, creeds call them what you will—have a common inspiration; we need no further proof than we have already received that no one of the many developments from the common source is in itself complete and perfect; there is good evidence that each new development as soon as it becomes specialized is separated from the true source, becomes over-elaborated, and so works its own downfall, the principle becoming absorbed and dominated by the bias of some individual mind—such is my analysis of the phenomena. It follows that what we seek is the noumenon, the reality, the true idea that underlies all these various manifestations.

Before I attempt to trace the common principle, however, I wish to make three statements.

(1) I do not profess to offer a finally perfected theory, for by so doing I should lay myself open to the same arguments I have advanced against standing other theories of the same nature. I say, frankly, that we are only at the beginnings of understanding, and my own wish is to keep my theory as simple as possible, to avoid any dogma.

(2) I do not propose in this place, for many reasons, to consider my own methods in any other connection but that of their application to physical defects, to the eradication of diseases, distortions, and lack of control, and,

24

progressively, to the science of race-culture and the improvement of the physique of the generations to come.

(3) I wish it to be clearly understood that this brochure is not finally definitive. I hope in the future to have many opportunities of examining the complexes, and of stating my experience of particular applications of my methods to peculiar cases, but I should not be true to my own principles if I were not willing to accept amendments, even, perhaps, to alter one or other of my premises should new facts tend to show that I have made a false assumption in any particular.

Now I have thus cleared the ground, I will examine what I believe to be the first and greatest stumbling-block to conscious self-control, namely, 'rigidity of mind,' which results in the fixed habit of thought and its concomitants— the functional and muscular habits passed on to sub-conscious control.

In defining rigidity of mind, I must hark back for a moment to that suggestive phrase of Mr. Trine's *In Tune with the Infinite*, though, in the present application, the rigidity I am concerned with is considered in a physical connection and does not involve interference with any non-spatial conceptions. It is rather the first half of the phase that is here of importance, for to be 'In Tune' conveys to my mind, and I wish it to convey the same meaning to others, the ideas of sensitiveness to impressions and responsiveness to the touch, when 'all the functions of life are becoming an intelligent harmony.' In a word, I want to suggest the idea of being open-minded, for even in reading this, if the individual deliberately puts himself in opposition to my point of view, he can by no possibility hope to benefit. Wherefore I desire, above all things, that he or she will read at least with an open mind and form no conclusion until I have finished, and will, perhaps, more particularly, subdue the interference of that great and ruling predisposition which has in the past so long impeded the advance of science.

Let us consider for a moment the application of rigidity of mind to physical functions. A person comes to me with some crippling defect due to the improper use of some organ or set of muscles. When I have diagnosed the defect and shown the patient *how* to use the organ or muscles in the proper way, I am always met at once with the reply, 'But I can't.' Let me ask any one who is reading this, and who suffers in any way, whether his or her attitude to the defect they suffer from is not precisely the same? Now this reply indicates directly that the control of the part affected is entirely sub-conscious; if it were not, we should merely have to substitute the hopeful 'I can' for that despondent 'I can't,' to remove the trouble. By (*a*) hypnotic treatment, by (*b*) faith-healing, or by (*c*) the application of the principles of the 'New Thought,' the patient in such a case would have the sub-conscious control influenced, either (*a*) by the mechanical means of trance and suggestion by the hypnotist, which leaves the conscious mind in exactly the original condition and merely changes (and it may be only temporarily) the habit of the sub-conscious control, or (*b* and *c*) by reiterated commands of the objective mind, perhaps heightened by the influencing suggestion of the healer or healers which, by repetition, substitute one habit for another without any apprehension by the intelligence or the true method of the exchange or, what is quite as frequent and far more harmful, shut out the sensitiveness to pain from the cerebral centres, and so leave the radical evil, no longer labelled by nature's warning, to work the patient's destruction in secret. Briefly, all three methods seek to reach the subjective mind by deadening the objective or conscious mind, and the centre and backbone of my theory and practice, which I feel that I cannot insist upon too strongly, is that THE CONSCIOUS MIND MUST BE QUICKENED.

It will be seen from this statement that my theory is in some ways a revolutionary one, since all earlier methods have in some form or another sought to put the flexible working of the true consciousness out of action in order to reach the sub-consciousness. The result of those methods it, logically and inevitably, to endeavour to alter a bad subjective habit and leave the objective habit of thought unchanged. The teachings of the 'New Thought' and many sects of faith-healers set out clearly enough that the patient must think rightly before he can be cured, but automatically, as it were, they then set about the carrying out of their teaching by prescribing 'affirmatives' or some sort of 'auto-suggestion' which are, in effect, no more than a kind of self-hypnotism, and, as such, are debasing to the primary functions of the intelligence.

I will take a simple instance from my own experience to illustrate a case in point.

A patient, whom I will call X, came to of me with an obstinate stammer arising from a congenital defect in the co-ordination of the face, tongue and throat muscles. Whenever X attempted to speak he drew down his upper lip. This was the outward sign of a series of vicious acts connected with a train of muscular movements; a sign that the ideo-motor centres were working to convey a wrong guiding influence to the specific parts concerned in the act of speech. These guiding influences rendered X quite incapable of speech, and would, indeed, have so prevented any other individual who produced the same working of the parts concerned. To insist in such a case that X should repeat 'I can speak,' or 'I won't stutter,' would be merely to endeavour to reach a supposed omniscient self-conscious self which would counteract the evil by the exercise of some assumed and separate intelligence possessed by it. I undertook the case by appealing to X's intelligence. Now, strange as it may seem (and I intend to treat this curious perversion in my next chapter), X's objective intelligence is not so easily reached and influenced as might appear.

He has formed a muscular habit of drawing down his lip independent of his conscious control, and the line of suggestion set up by the wish to speak induces at once a reflex action of a complicated set of muscles. X has learned to do this automatically and at first seems incapable of controlling those lip muscles when the wish to speak is initiated.

In this case my first endeavour must be directed to keeping in abeyance, by the power of inhibition, all the mental associations connected with the idea of speaking; and to eradicating all erroneous, pre-conceived ideas concerning the things X imagines he can or cannot do or what is or it not possible. My next effort must be to give X correct and conscious control of all the parts concerned, including, of course, the lip and face muscles, preparatory to the very conception of speaking during the practice of the exercises, and to get this control he must have a complete and perfect apprehension of all the muscles concerned. In originating some new idea which is to take the place of the old idea of drawing down the upper lip, it may be necessary at first to break the old association by some new order, such as deliberately to draw the lip up, to open the mouth, or to make some similar muscular act previously unfamiliar in its application to the act of speech. The new order is then substituted for the command to speak. X is told not to speak but to draw up his lip, open his mouth, etc. It will be understood that I have omitted much detail touching the interdependence of the parts concerned, but I wish here to convey only the essentials of method rather than the physiological explanation of their working. It must always be remembered that Nature works as a whole and not in parts, and once the true cause of the evil is discovered and eradicated, all the affected mechanisms can soon be restored to their full capacity. I may note here that X was completely cured of his stammer, and that his was a particularly obstinate case, a fact chiefly due to the confirmation of a wrong habit in early childhood.

This is an example, chosen for its simplicity, to illustrate the prime essentials of my theory, but it is capable of a very wide application, so wide that it may be applied to the working not only of the ordinary controlled muscles, but of the semi-automatic muscles which actuate the vital organs. Not many years ago an Indian Yogi was examined by Professor Max Müller at Cambridge, and we have it on the authority of the latter that this Yogi was able to stop the beating of his own heart at will and suffer no harmful consequences.

Let it be clearly understood, however that I have no sympathy with these abnormal manifestations, which I regard as a dangerous trickery practised on the body, a trickery in no way admirable or to be sought after. The performances of the Yogis do not certainly command my admiration, and the well-known system of breathing practised and taught by them is, in my opinion, not only wrong and essentially crude, but tends also to exaggerate those very defects from which we suffer in this twentieth century. I have merely quoted this case of the Yogi in support of my assertion that there is no function of the body that cannot be brought under the control of the conscious will.

That this is, indeed a fact and not a theory, I do claim without hesitation, and I claim further that by the application of this principle of conscious control there may, in time, be evolved a complete mastery over the body, which will result in elimination of all physical defects. Certain aspects of this control and the reasons why it has not been acquired, I will treat under the next heading.

V.
HABITS OF THOUGHT AND OF BODY

'The man who has so far made up his mind about anything that he can no longer reckon freely with that thing, is mad where that thing is concerned.' — ALLEN UPWARD, *The New Word*

WHEN speaking of the case of stammering cited in my last chapter, I had occasion to note that it was not an easy task to influence X's conscious mind. The point is this; a patient who submits himself for treatment, whether to a medical man or to any other practitioner, may DO what he is told, but will not or cannot THINK as he is told. In ordinary practice, the man who has taken a medical degree disregards this mental attitude in ninety-nine cases out of a hundred. Medicine, diet, or exercise is prescribed, and if the patient obediently follows the mechanical directions given with regard to the prescriptions, he is considered a good patient. The doctor does not trouble as to the patient's attitude of mind, except in that one case out of a hundred, possibly a case of flagrant hypochondria.

Indeed I am willing to maintain and prove in this connection that a very large percentage of cases which are now being treated in our public and private lunatic asylums, have been allowed to develop insanity by reason of this disregard of the mental attitude. I cannot stop now to consider this interesting subject of insanity, but I must note in passing that that very large percentage of the cases I have mentioned, should never have been allowed to arrive at the condition which made it necessary to send them to an asylum in the first instance. Very many of them, so far from lacking mental control, are minds of quite exceptional ability, among them being instances of subjects who have assumed a deliberate attitude in the first place to subserve a private end, such as the avoidance of uncongenial work, or the over-indulgence of some desire or perverted sense, though the attitude which was first adopted deliberately, became afterwards a fixed habit, and so uncontrollable.

29

When we are seeking to give a patient conscious control, the consideration of mental attitude, therefore, must precede the performance of the act prescribed. The act performed is of less consequence than the manner of its performance. And yet, though the patient or inquirer into the system may apprehend this fact, he often finds an enormous difficulty in altering some trifling habit of thought which stands between him and the benefit he clearly expects.

The truth of the matter is that the majority of people fall into a mechanical habit of thought as easily as they fall into the mechanical habit of body which is the immediate consequence.

I will take an instance from a subject outside my own province in order to bring the matter home; but I will preface my illustration by pointing out that I, personally, am not in the least concerned to alter the habit of thought of either of the persons I adduce as an example, and only cite well-known political propaganda in order to give vividness to my picture.

Let us suppose then that A is a convinced Free-trader, and that Z is no less certain of the glorious possibilities of Protection and let us set A and Z to argue the matter. We notice at once that when A is speaking Z's endeavours are confined to catching him in a misstatement or in a fault of logic, and A's attitude is precisely the same when Z holds the stage. Neither partisan has the least intention from the outset of altering his creed, nor could either be convinced by the facts and arguments of the other, however sound. This is a fact within the experience of every intelligent person. The disputants have so influenced their own minds that they are incapable of receiving certain impressions; a part of their intelligence normally susceptible of receiving new ideas, even if such ideas are opposed to earlier conceptions, is in a state of anæsthesia; it is shut off, put out of action. The habit of mind which has been formed mechanically translates all the arguments of an opponent into misconceptions or fallacies. Neither disputant in our illustration has the least intention or desire to approach the subject with an open mind. Unfortunately, the rigid habit of mind does not only apply to the issues of government; it is evidenced in all the thoughts and acts of our daily life, and is the cause of many demonstrable evils.

Returning now to my own province of therapeutics, I need hardly instance any special example to carry my point. Of late years much attention has been given to the consideration of the mental attitude with regard to disease, and though no clearly defined remedy has been advanced, the condition has been diagnosed and defined. The 'fixed idea,' hallucination, obsession, are all terms used deliberately to denote a morbid condition, but we have to apply these terms much more widely and grasp the fact that they are applicable to small, disregarded mental habits as well as to the well-defined evils which marked their development. In the case of X, the mental habit which had grown up as the result of postulating 'I can't draw my lip up before speaking,' was only another aspect of the attitude of A and Z towards the subject of their discussion, and it was precisely similar in kind. The aggregate of these habits is so characteristic in some cases that we see how easily the fallacy arose of assuming an entity for the sub-conscious self, a self which at the last analysis is made up of those acquired habits and of certain other habits (some of them labelled instincts) the predisposition to which is our birthright, a predisposition inherited from that long chain of ancestors whose origin goes back to the first dim emergence of active life. Fortunately for us there is not a single one of these habits of mind, with their resultant habits of body, which may not be altered by the inculcation of those principles concerning the true poise of the body which I have called the principles of mechanical advantage,[12] used in co-operation with an understanding of the inhibitory and volitional powers of the objective mind; by which means these deterrent habits can be raised to conscious control. The false pose and carriage of the body; the incorrect and laboured habits of breathing that are the cause of many troubles besides the obvious ill-effects on the lungs and heart; the degeneration of the muscular system; the partial failure of many vital organs; the morbid, fatty conditions that destroy the semblance of men and women to human beings;—all these things and many more that combine to cause disability, disease, and death, are the result of incorrect habits of mind and body, all of which may be changed into correct and beneficial habits if once we can clear away that first impeding habit of thought which stands between us and conscious control.

I believe I have at last laid myself quite open to the attack of the habitual objector, a person I am really anxious to conciliate. I have given him the

---

[12] Certain aspects of these principles will be found set out in the two pamphlets which I have incorporated in this volume.

opportunity of pointing a finger at my last paragraph and saying, 'But you only want to change one habit for another. If, as you have implied, the habit of mind is bad, why encourage habits at all, even if they are as you say, "correct and beneficial"?'

This is a point of the first importance. But in the first place it is essential to understand the difference between the habit that is recognized and understood, and the habit that is not. The difference in its application to the present case is that the first can be altered at will and the second cannot. For once real conscious control is obtained, a 'habit' need never be fixed; it is not truly a habit at all, but an order or series of orders given to the subordinate controls of the body, which orders will be carried out until countermanded.

Let us consider for a moment the import of this statement. Suppose a patient comes to me who has acquired incorrect respiratory habits, and suppose that he is plastic and ready to assimilate new methods, and that he soon learns consciously to make a proper use of the muscular mechanism which governs the movements of the breathing apparatus, a word that fitly describes this particular mechanism of the body. Now it would be absurd to suppose that thereafter this person should in his waking moments deliberately apprehend each separate working of his lungs. He has acquired conscious control of that working, it is true, but once, that control has been mastered, the actual movements that follow are given in charge of the 'sub-conscious self,' but always on the understanding that a counter order may be given at any moment if necessary. Until such counter order is given, however, if it ever need be given, the working of the lungs is for all intents and purposes sub-conscious, though it may be elevated to the level of the conscious at any moment. Thus it will be seen that the difference between the new habit and the old is that the old was our master and ruled us, while the new is our servant ready to carry out our lightest wish without question, though always working quietly and unobtrusively on our behalf in accordance with the most recent orders given.

Briefly, as I see it, the sub-consciousness in this application is only a synonym for that rigid routine we finally refer to as habit; this rigid routine being the stumbling-block to rapid adaptability, to the assimilation of new ideas, to originality. On the other hand, the consciousness is the synonym for mobility of mind, for all that the sub-conscious control checks and impedes, a mobility which will obtain for us physical regeneration and a mental outlook that will open new and wider possibilities in the enjoyment of those powers we all possess, but which are so often deliberately stunted or neglected.

Consider this point also in its application to the case of John Doe, cited in my second chapter. If the mental attitude of hypothetical individual had been changed, and he had learned to use his muscles consciously; if, instead of automatically performing a set of muscle-tensing exercises, he had devoted himself to apprehending the control of his muscles and the co-ordination of them, he could have carried his knowledge into every act of his life. In his most sedentary occupations he could have been using and exercising his muscular system without resort to any violent contortions, waving of the arms or kicking of the legs; and I cannot but think that in the first place he could better have employed those hours spent in this manner by taking a walk in the open air or by occupying himself with some other form of natural exercise. Still, if in his case certain mild forms of exercise at certain times were necessary, such exercises should have used and employed his mental and physical powers, and through those agencies should have used his muscular mechanism in such a way that its uses could have been applied to the simplest acts, such as sitting on a stool and writing at a desk. There would then have been no question of what we termed civil war within the body; the whole physical machinery would have been co-ordinated and adapted to John Doe's way of life.

In an earlier paragraph I pointed out that John Doe was suffering from certain mental and physical delusions, and I endeavoured to show how those delusions militated against his recovery of health. Returning to this point now that the correct method has been indicated, I may use his case to give another example of this method. What John Doe lacked was a conscious and proper recognition of the right uses of the parts of his muscular mechanism, since while he still uses such parts wrongly, the performance of physical exercises will only increase the defects. He will, in fact, merely copy some other person in the performance of a particular exercise; copy him in the outward act, while his own consciousness of the act performed and the means and uses of his muscular mechanism will remain unaltered. Therefore, before he attempts any form of physical development, he must discover, or find someone who can discover for him, what are his defects in the uses indicated. When this has been done he must, proceed to inhibit the guiding sensations which cause him to use the mechanism imperfectly, apprehend the position of mechanical advantage, and then by using the new, correct guiding sensations or orders, he will be able to bring about the proper use of his muscular mechanism with perfect ease. If the mechanical principle employed is a correct one, every movement will be made with a minimum of effort, and he will not be conscious of the slightest tension. In time will follow a recognition of the new and correct use of the mechanism, which use will then become established and be employed in the acts of everyday life.

For instance, if we decide that a defect must be got rid of or a mode of action changed, and if we proceed in the ordinary way directly to eradicate it, we shall fail invariably, and with reason. Should a man habitually stiffen his neck in walking, sitting, or other ordinary acts of life, it evidences that he is endeavouring to do with the muscles of his neck the work which should be performed by certain other muscles of his body, notably those of the back. Now it follows that if he is told to relax those stiffened muscles of the neck and obeys the order, this mere act of relaxation deals only with an effect, and does not quicken his consciousness of the use of the right mechanism which he should use in place of those relaxed. The desire to stiffen the neck muscles should be inhibited as a preliminary (which is not the same thing at all as a direct order to relax the muscles themselves), and then the true uses of the muscular mechanism, the means of placing the body in a position of mechanical advantage, must be studied, when the work will naturally devolve on those muscles intended to carry it out, and the neck will be relaxed unconsciously. The conscious orders in this case, the orders given to the right muscles, are preventative orders, and the due sequence of cause and effect is maintained.

But the full discussion of the principles of physical culture must be left to a later work,[13] and I will, here, only note one more point in concluding my reference to the hypothecated John Doe, who, nevertheless, stands as the representative of a very large body of people. This point is the question of the storing and reserving of energy, and what I may call, to use a phrase which has a mechanical equivalent, the registration of tension. If you ask a man to lift a papier-maché imitation of an enormous dumb-bell, leading him to believe

---

[13] See also the two pamphlets incorporated in this volume, viz. 'A New Method of Respiratory Vocal Re-education' and 'Re-education of the Kinæsthetic Systems.'

that it is almost beyond his capacity to raise it from the floor, he will exert his full power in the effort to do that which he could perform with the greatest ease. In a lesser degree the same expenditure of unnecessary force is exerted by the vast majority of 'physical-culture' students, and by practically every person in the ordinary duties of daily life. The mind has not been taught to register correctly the tension, or, in other words, to gauge accurately the amount of muscular effort required to perform certain acts, the expenditure of effort always being in excess of what is required, an excellent instance of the lack of harmony in the untutored organism. This fact may be easily tested by any interested person who will take the trouble to try its application. Ask a friend to lift a chair or any other weight such that while it may be lifted without great difficulty, it will in the process make an undoubted call on the muscular energies. You will see at once that your friend will approach the task with a definite preconception as to the amount of physical tension necessary, Before ever he has approached it, he will brace or tense the muscles of his arms, back, neck, etc., and when about to perform the act he will place himself in a position which is one of mechanical disadvantage so far as he is concerned. All these preparations are, of course, quite unnecessary, but the whole attitude of mind towards the task is wrong; in this instance, indeed, any preconception as to the degree of tension required is out of place. If we desire to lift a weight with the least possible waste of energy, we should approach it and grasp it with relaxed muscles, assuming the position of greatest possible mechanical advantage, and then gradually exert our muscular energies until sufficient power is attained to overcome the resistance.

Returning now to the consideration of that bias or predisposing habit of mind which so often balks us at the outset, we may see at once that this predisposition takes many curious forms. Sometimes it is frankly objective, and is outlined in the statement, 'Well, I don't believe in all this, but I may as well try it.' In this form a single unlocked-for result is generally enough to change disbelief into credulity. I write the word 'credulity' with intention, for I mean to imply that the reaction in a certain to type of mind is little, if any, better than the profession of disbelief. What is required is not prejudice in either direction, but a calm, clear, open-eyed intelligence, a ready, adaptive outlook, believe me, which does not connote indefiniteness of purpose or uncertainty of initiative.

Another form of predisposition arises from lack of purpose, and the mental habits that go with this condition are hard to eradicate, more particularly when the original feebleness has led to some form of hypochondria or nervous disease which has been treated with the usual disregard of the radical evil. It is not difficult for the most superficial inquirer to understand that any method of treating the subject still further of the exercise of initiative—such a method is the rest cure, for instance, though I could quote many others—only increases the original evil. The lack of purpose is pandered to and cultivated; and after the six weeks or so of treatment the patient returns to his or her duties in ordinary life, even more unfitted than before to perform them. As I have said before, no account is taken of the instinct for self-preservation or the will to live. This is the very mainspring of human life, yet a power which in the routine of protected civilization tends at times to become relaxed, and so the machinery runs down. Then the machinery must be wound up again, not allowed to become still further relaxed by resting. And this lack of purpose—the immediate effect of our educational methods—is, unhappily, very common in all classes, but especially among those who have no occupation and those whose employment is a mechanical routine which does not exercise the powers of initiative. The curious thing about this very large class is that they do not really want to be cured. They may be suffering from many physical disabilities or from actual physical pain, and they may and will protest most earnestly that they want to be free from those pains and disabilities, but in the face of the evidence we must admit that if the objective wish is really there, it is so feeble as to be non-existent for all practical purposes. In many cases this attitude of submission to illness is the outcome of a strong subjective habit. The trouble, whatever it is, is endured in the first instance; it is looked upon as a nuisance, perhaps, but not as an intolerable nuisance; no steps are taken to be rid of it, and the trouble grows and, by degrees, is looked upon as a necessity. Then, at last, when the trouble has increased until it threatens the interruption of all ordinary occupations, the sufferer seeks a remedy, but the habit of submission has grown too strong, and while the disease can be kept within certain bounds, no effort is made to fight it. This is, of course, one of the commonest experiences in the healing profession. A patient is treated and benefited, and seems on the high-road to perfect health. Then follows a relapse. The first question put is 'Have you been following the treatment?' and the answer, if the patient is truthful, is, 'I forgot,' or 'I didn't bother any more about it.' In a recent experience of a medical friend of mine, a patient confessed to having stayed in the house for a week after a certain relapse occurred, although the very essence of the prescription by which he had previously benefited was to be in the fresh air as much as possible. This simply means that the subjective habit of submission has grown too strong for the objective mind—weakened in its turn by the neglect of its guiding functions—to conquer. No prescription or course of treatment can have any effect upon such a patient as this, unless that subjective habit can be brought within the sphere of conscious control. In other cases this apparent lack of desire for health is due to an attachment to some dearly loved habit, which must be given up if the proper functions of the body are to be resumed. It may be a habit of small self-indulgence or one that is imminently threatening the collapse of the vital processes, but the attachment to it is so strong, that the enfeebled objective mind prefers to hold to the habit and risk death sooner than make the effort of opposing it. Yet even in cases where no harm can be traced directly to a markedly influencing habit, the general, all-pervading habit of lassitude or inertia is so strong that any regime which may be prescribed is distasteful if it involves, as it must, the exercise of those powers which have been allowed to fall more or less into disuse.

Space will not permit of my instancing further examples of the predisposing habit, but very little introspection on the part of my readers should enable them to diagnose their own peculiar mental habits, the first step towards being rid of them. We must always remember that the vast majority of human beings live very narrow lives, doing the same thing, and thinking the same thoughts day by day; and it is this very fact that makes it so necessary that we should acquire conscious control of the mental and physical powers as a whole, for we otherwise run the risk of losing that versatility which is such an essential factor in their development.

If, after reading so far, they feel inclined to analyze these habits and to set about a control of them, I will give them one word of preliminary advice, 'Beware of so-called concentration!'

This advice is so pertinent to the whole principle that it is worth while to elaborate it. Ask any one you know to concentrate his mind on a subject—

anything will do, a place, a person, or a thing. If your friend is willing to play the game and earnestly endeavours to concentrate his mind, he will probably knit his forehead, tense his muscles, clench his hands, and either close his eyes or stare fixedly at some point in the room. As a result his mind is very fully occupied with this unusual condition of the body, which can only be maintained by repeated orders from the objective mind. In short, your friend, though he may not know it, is not using his mind for the consideration of the subject you have given him to concentrate upon, but for the consideration of an unusual bodily condition which he calls concentration. This is true, also, of the attitude of *attention* required for children in schools; it dissociates the brain instead of compacting it. Personally, I do not believe in any concentration which calls for effort. It is the wish, the conscious desire to do a thing or think a thing, which results in adequate performance. Could Spencer have written his *First Principles*, or Darwin his *Descent of Man*, if either had been forced to any rigid narrowing effort in order to keep his mind on the subject in hand? I do net deny that some work can be done under conditions which desire or necessitate such an artificially arduous effort, but I do deny that it is ever the best work. Now I will admit that such a case as that of Sir Walter Scott can logically be argued against this view. For the real earnest wish to write the Waverley novels was there, even if it originated in the desire to pay the debts he took upon himself, and not in the desire to write the novels because he took a pleasure in the actual performance. Briefly, our application of the word 'concentration' denotes conflict which is a morbid condition and a form of illness; singleness of purpose is quite another thing. If you try to straighten your arm and bend it at the same moment, you may exercise considerable muscular effort, but you will achieve no result, and the analogy applies to the endeavour to delimit the powers of the brain by concentration, and at the same time to exercise them to the full extent. The endeavour represents the conflict of two postulates, 'I must' and 'I can't'; the fight continues indefinitely, with a constant waste of misapplied effort. Once eradicate the mental habit of thinking that this effort is necessary, once postulate and apprehend the meaning of 'I wish' instead of these former contradictions, and what was difficult will become easy, and pleasure will be substituted for pain. We must cultivate, in brief, the deliberate habit of taking up every occupation with the whole mind, with a living desire to carry each action through to a successful accomplishment, a desire which necessitates bringing into play every faculty of the attention. By use, the power develops, and it soon becomes as simple to alter a morbid taste which may have been a lifelong tendency as to alter the smallest of recently acquired bad habits.

In all these efforts to apprehend and control mental habits, the first and only real difficulty is to overcome the preliminary inertia of mind in order to combat the subjective habit. The brain becomes used to thinking in a certain way, it works in a groove, and when actuated, slides along the familiar, well-worn path; but if once it is lifted, as it were, it is astonishing how easily it may be directed. At first it will have a tendency to return to the old groove and work as before by means of one mechanical, unintelligent operation, but the groove soon fills, and though, thereafter, we may be able to use the old path if we choose, we are no longer bound to it.

In concluding this brief note on mental habits I turn my attention particularly to the many who say, 'I am quite content as I am.' To them I say, firstly, if you are content to be the slave of habits instead of master of your own mind and body, you have never realized the wonderful inheritance which is yours by right of the fact that you were born a reasoning, intelligent man or woman. But, I say, secondly, and this is of importance to the larger world, and is not confined to your intimate circle, 'What of the children?' Are you content to rob them of their inheritance, as, perhaps, you were robbed by your parents? Are you willing to send them out into the world ill-equipped; dependent on precepts and incipient habits; unable to control their own desires, and already well on the way to physical degeneration? Happily, I believe that the means of stirring the inert is being provided. The question of Eugenics—or the science of race culture—is being debated by earnest men and women; and the whole problem of contemporary physical degeneration is one which looms ever larger in the public mind. It is the problem which has exercised me for many years, and which is mainly responsible for the issue of this brochure, and in my next chapter I shall treat it in connection with the theory of progressive conscious control which I have outlined in the foregoing pages.

VI.
RACE CULTURE AND THE TRAINING OF THE CHILDREN

'In what way to treat the body; in what way to treat the mind; in what way to manage our affairs; in what way to bring up a family; in what way to behave as a citizen; in what way to utilize those sources of happiness which nature supplies—how to use all our faculties to the greatest advantage; how to live completely? And this being the great thing needful for us to learn, is, by consequence, the great thing which education has to teach. To prepare us for complete living is the function which education has to discharge.' — HERBERT SPENCER, *Education*

EVERY child is born into the world with a predisposition to certain habits. For many months, the period varying with the sex and ability of the infant, its vital processes and movements are for all practical purposes independent of any conscious control, and the human infant remains in this helpless, dependent condition much longer than any other animal. The habits which the child evidences during this protracted period are those hereditary predispositions which are early developed by circumstance and environment, habits of muscular uses, vital functioning, and of adaptability. If it were possible to analyze the tendencies of a child when it is, say, twelve months old, we could soon master the science of heredity, which is at present so tentative and uncertain in its deductions, but the child's potentialities lie hidden in the mysterious groupings and arrangement of its cells and tissues; hid beyond the reach of any analysis. The child is our material; within certain wide limits we may mould it into the shape we desire. But even at birth it is differentiated from other children; though our limits may be wide, they are fixed; nevertheless, within those limits our capacity for good and evil is very great.

There are two methods by which a child learns. The first, and in earlier years the predominant, method is by imitation; the second is by, precept or directly administered instruction, positive or negative.

With regard to the first method, parents of every class will admit the fact not only that children imitate those who are with them during those early, plastic years, but that the child's first efforts to, assimilate itself to the conditions surrounding it are based almost exclusively on imitation. For, despite the many thousand years during which some form of civilization has been in existence, no child has yet been born into the world with hereditary instincts tending to fit it for any particular society. Its language and manners, for instance, are modelled entirely on the speech and habits of those who have charge of it; the child descended from a hundred kings will speak the language and adopt the manners of the East End should it be reared among these associations; and the son of an Australian aboriginal would speak the English tongue and behave as a civilized child if brought up with English people.

No one denies this fact, it has been proved and accepted, yet we never seek to make a practical application of our knowledge. The science of heredity is still tentative and indeterminate, but no reasoning person can doubt from this and other instances that in the vast majority of cases, at least, the influence of heredity can be practically eradicated. Personally I see very clearly, from facts of my own observation, that when the characteristics of the father and mother are analyzed, and their faults and virtues understood, a proper training of the children will prevent the same faults and encourage the same virtues in their children.

To appreciate to the utmost the effect of training upon the children, we must remember that the first tastes, likes, or dislikes of the infant begin to be developed during the first two or three days after birth. Long before the infant is a month old, habits, tending to become fixed habits, have been developed, and if these habits are not harmful, well and good. The first sense developed is the sense of taste, a sense that develops very quickly and needs the most careful attention. Artificial feeding is in itself a very serious danger, but when this feeding is in the hands of careless or ignorant persons the danger becomes increased a hundredfold. An instance of this is the common idea that considerable quantities of sugar should be added to the milk. This is done very often to induce the child to take food against its natural desire. It may be that the child has been suffering from some slight internal derangement, and Nature's remedy has been to affect the child with a distaste for food in order to give the stomach a rest. Then the unthinking mother tempts the child with sugar, and all sorts of internal trouble may follow. But in such a case as this the taste for a particular thing, such as sugar, is encouraged, and apart from the direct harm which may result, the habit becomes the master of the child, and may rule it through life; the child, in fact, is sent out into the world the slave of the sense of taste.

Unfortunately, in ninety cases out of a hundred, children up to the age of six or seven years are allowed to acquire very decided tastes for things which are harmful. Women are not trained for the sphere of motherhood, do not give these matters the thought and attention they deserve, and hence they do not understand the most elementary principles concerning the future welfare of their offspring in such matters as feeding and sense guidance. Children are net taught to cultivate a taste for wholesome, nourishing foods, but are tempted, and their incipient habits pandered to, by such additions as the sugar I have more particularly cited.

At the present time I know a child of five years old whose taste is already perverted by the method, or lack of method, I have indicated. The child dislikes milk unless undue quantities of sugar are added, will not eat such food as milk puddings or brown bread, and has a strong distaste for cream. It is almost impossible to make the child eat vegetables of any kind, but he is always ready to take large quantities of meat and sweets. The child is already suffering from malnutrition and serious internal derangement. The latter would be greatly improved by small quantities of olive oil taken daily, but it is only with the greatest difficulty that he can be induced to take it. If the child lives with his parents for the next ten years, he will grow into a weak and ailing boy, and will suffer from the worst forms of digestive trouble and imperfect functioning of the internal organs.

Apropos of this point, I remember hearing a question put to my friend, Dr. Clubbe of Sydney, by a London specialist, who asked what, in Dr. Clubbe's opinion, was the primary cause of the derangement of the natural working of a child's muscular mechanism and respiratory system. The answer was given without hesitation. 'Toxic poisoning as a result of artificial feeding.' The logic of this answer will be readily apprehended by the layman when he considers the interdependence of every part of the system, for in this case the nerve centres connected with the sensory apparatus of the digestive organs and the urea control also the respiratory processes. As a consequence, when these centres are dulled in their action as a result of toxic poisoning, there is a loss of activity in the processes of respiration, with consequent readjustments of those parts of the muscular mechanism more nearly concerned, and so the whole machine is thrown out of gear.

Thus we see that in such instances the mischief begins very early in the life of the child, and it is carried on and exaggerated with every step in its development. Even in babyhood precept or coercion comes into play. When the child cries, little effort is made to discover the cause. Often the child is soothed by being carried up and down the room. It is wonderful how soon the infant begins to associate some rudiments of cause and effect; the child who is unduly pandered to will soon learn to cry whenever it desires to be rocked or dandled, and thus the foundations of pandering to sensation are quickly laid.

But as the child comes to the observant age its habits begin to grow more quickly. We have admitted that a child imitates its parents or nurses in tricks of manner and speech, yet we do not stop to consider that it will also imitate our carriage of the body, our performance of muscular acts, even our very manner of breathing. It is a wonderful force this faculty for imitation and adaptation, one which we majority have at our command if we would only pause to consider how we may use it in the right way. The vast of wrong habits acquired by children result from their imitation of the imperfect models confronting them. But how many parents attempt to put a right model before their children? How learn to eradicate their own defects of pose and carriage, so that they may be better examples to the child? How many in choosing a nurse will take the trouble to select a girl whom they would like their children to imitate? Very, very few, and the reason is simple. In the first place they do not realize the harmful effect of bad example, and in the second the great majority of the parents have so little perception of truth in this matter that they are incapable of choosing a girl who is a good specimen of humanity, and are sublimely unconscious of their own crookedness and defects. What then can we hope from these parents who are, at the present time, so unfit, so incapable of teaching their own children the primer of physical life? And I may note here that this principle has a wider application than that of the nursery; it holds, also, in connection with the model of physical well-being set by the teachers in all primary and secondary schools. There is no need for me to elaborate this theme; the iniquity of allowing children to be trained in physical exercises—in our Board schools, for instance—by a teacher who is obviously physically unfit, is sufficiently glaring.

The crux of the whole question is that we are progressing towards conscious control, and have not yet realized all that this progress connotes. Children, as civilization becomes continually more the natural condition, evince fewer and fewer of their original, savage instincts. In early life they are dependent more and more upon their instructors and less upon sub-conscious direction. The child of the present day, once it has emerged from its first state of absolute helplessness, and before it has been trained and coerced into certain mental and physical habits, is the most plastic and adaptable of living things. It has at this stage the complete potentiality of conscious control which are to be developed by the eradication of certain hereditary tendencies or predispositions, but the usual procedure is to thrust certain habits upon it, without the least consideration of cause and effect, and insist upon these habits until they have become sub-conscious and passed from the region of intellectual guidance.

I will take one instance as an example of this—the point of right- and left-handed ness. We assume from the outset, and the superstition is so old that its source is untraceable, that a child must learn to depend upon its right hand, and despise the use of its left. This superstition has so sunk into our minds by repetition that it has become incorporated in our language. 'Dexterous' stands for an admirable, and 'sinister' for an inauspicious, quality; and we may even find ignorant people at the present day who say that they would never trust a left-handed person. As a result of this attitude and of the absolute rule laid down, that a child must learn to write and use its knife with the right hand only, the number of ambidextrous people is limited to the few who, by some initial accident, used their left hand by preference, and were afterwards taught to use their right. In a fairly wide experience I do not remember to have heard of a father or mother who has said 'this child may become an artist or a pianist,' for example, 'and may therefore need to develop the sensitiveness and powers of manipulation of the left hand as well as the right'; though I have known many cases where much time and trouble had to be expended in acquiring the uses of the left hand later in life; such cases as those of persons suffering from writers' cramp, and dependent for their living on their ability to use a pen.

I have cited this example of right-handedness because it exhibits the pliability of the physical mechanism in early life and the manner in which we thoughtlessly bind it to some method of working, without ever stopping to think whether that method is good in itself, or whether it is the one best adapted for the conditions of life into which the child will grow. We thrust a rigid rule of physical life and mental outlook upon the children. We are not convinced that the rule is the best, or even that it is a good rule; often we know, or would know if we gave the matter a moment's consideration, that in our own bodies the rule has not worked particularly well; but it is the rule which was taught to us, and we pass it on by precept, and by holding up our imperfections for imitation, and then wonder what is the cause of our present physical degeneration.

In this note on race culture and the training of children, I have thus far dwelt almost exclusively on the earlier years of childhood; but I have much to say at some future time on the questions of primary and secondary education; of the boy and girl at school between the ages of, say, seven and eighteen. No one who has read this brochure with attention, and earnestly attempted to comprehend my point of view, will now be able to urge that the question of education, secular or religious, is outside my province, but, at the risk of being accused of repetition, I will state my case in this connection once again, briefly, as follows:

The mental and physical are so inextricably combined that we cannot regard one without the other. In this matter of education I am, admittedly, an iconoclast. I would fain break down the idols of tradition and set up new concepts. In no matters do we see more plainly the harmful effect of the rigid convention than in this matter of teaching. We speak commonly of training the minds of children. It is a happy expression in its origin, and we still retain its proper intention when we apply the word to its uses in horticulture. The gardener does, indeed, train the young growth, draws it out to the light and warmth, leads it into the conditions most helpful for its development.

But when we speak of training a child we never intend that we wish to draw it out, to let it expand and develop; we mean, on the contrary, that we wish to repress it mentally, to cut and twist it into strange shapes, and repress and stunt it, in order that it may grow into the narrow, warped, blind shape into which we also were forced as children.

In teaching, the first essential is to cultivate the uses of the mind and body, and not, as is ordinarily the case, to neglect the instruments of thought and reason by the inculcation of fixed rules which have never been examined. Again, where ideas that are patently erroneous have already been formed, the teacher should take pains to apprehend these preconceptions, and in dealing with them should not attempt to overlay them, but to eradicate them as far as possible before teaching or submitting the new and correct idea. I say 'teaching or submitting,' and perhaps the latter word better expresses my meaning, for by teaching I understand the placing of facts, for and against, before the child in such a way as to appeal to his reasoning faculties, and to his latent powers of originality. He should be allowed to think for himself, and should not be crammed with other people's ideas, or one side only of a controversial subject. Why should not the child's powers of intelligence be trained? Why should they be stunted by forcing him to accept the preconceived ideas and traditions which have been handed down from generation to generation, without examination, without reason, without inquiry as to their truth or origin. The human mind of to-day is suffering partial paralysis by this method of forcing these unreasoned and antiquated principles upon the young and plastic intelligence. The educational system, itself, is grievously inadequate and detrimental, as all thinking educationalists are aware, but the decision regarding the necessity for physical exercise and 'deep-breathing' in our schools has added another evil. It is only necessary to study intelligently the work recently issued by the Education Department, in order to recognize the truth of this statement, and I intend in the near future to deal with that publication and demonstrate the effects of applying the principles and exercises embodied in it, for I am convinced that nothing can result from their application but complete chaos, physical and mental.

To return to my general theory of training, I fear I must not particularize too definitely in some directions, but my instance of right-handedness has its application. What is our own creed or convention? Have we ever examined any detail of it by the light of our reason, tested it in its application to life and knowledge? Not in one case out of a thousand, but we still believe ourselves to be reasoning creatures, and if our child should discover a trace of intelligence and originality, if he or she should question for one moment the infallibility of the law binding the parent, the law which parent or schoolmaster has never dared to question, then the rod descends on the unhappy child, and you insist that the child should believe that you are right beyond question, each and every one of you undeniably, perpetually, infallibly right. But my client is the child, and on his behalf I plead that he may be allowed to choose, to exercise his reason and judgment, and expand the powers of his intelligence; for I know that when you limit him, when you bind him to fixed ideas, narrow his mind, and impart to him, deliberately, your own mental habits—despite the fact that you, yourselves, have never reasoned the matter, but have accepted what was given you without question—I know that when you do this you unwittingly stereotype him in other ways. The children, the youths, the adults whom I want, are those with open minds, for these may be trained in the best sense of the word to an ideal of physical and mental completeness. I would repeat and emphasize the concluding sentences of Mr. Allen Upward's delightful work, *The New Word*, which I have already quoted, and say with him, 'Give the child leave to grow. Give the child leave to live. Give the child leave to hope and to hope truly.... He is the plaintiff in this case. I say that he is mankind...and his birthright is the truth.'

It is full time that we gave more earnest thought to this matter. I cannot in this brief outline dwell on the many phases of proper food, clothing, and physical training, and all those other points which we must consider, and that immediately. But I have very much to say on the subject, and hope to have an opportunity in the near future of elaborating my methods and of setting them out so that they may be practically and universally applied. But if by these few remarks I can rouse some interest in this world problem, I shall have done something towards its solution. It is a problem which is very urgent at the present time, and is growing more urgent every day. All that we have done up to the present time is to enforce one or other rule upon the children as an experiment. For all the rules have been rigid in their enforcement, however unscientific in their conception. In place of these rules I look for an ideal which I believe to be comparatively easy of realization. I look for, and already see, a method of training our children which shall make them masters of their own bodies; I look for a time when the child shall be so taught and trained that whatever the circumstance which shall later surround it, it will without effort be able to adapt itself to its environment and be enabled to live its life in the enjoyment of perfect health, physical and mental.

VII.
A POSTSCRIPT

I HAD completed my first draft of this little brochure, and was engaged in making certain corrections and additions to it, when I received the number of the *British Medical Journal,* dated June 18, 1910. The contents of that number are almost exclusively devoted to the consideration of Mental- and Faith-healing, and articles are contributed by such well-known English medical men as Sir Clifford Allbutt, Sir Henry Morris, H.T. Butlin, and William Osler. The coincidence was remarkable, for I found in this issue an epitome of the general attitude towards mental therapeutics, ranging from a conception which I can only regard as primitive to the most detached and scientific analysis, but the real point of the coincidence was found in a review of a fifty-eight page brochure,[14] by a German professor, a brochure which also formed the subject of a leading article. Very little study of this number of the *British Medical Journal* was necessary to convince me that I must devote another chapter to its consideration, for it came as a most apt confirmation of the whole tendency of my work and writing, and will now serve to illustrate the fact that even the most academic of professions is slowly groping its way in the direction I have endeavoured to indicate in this work without the encumbrance of that involved language and those modes of thought with which the scientific writer cautiously cloaks his expression. Moreover, the daily press commented on this symposium of medical opinion, in many cases at some length, and I was not surprised to find that the comparatively lucid methods of journalism required that the writers should in some instances demand an explanation of the general tendency of these medical expressions, and were strongly inclined to ask why, if undoubted cures had been acknowledged, some attempt had not been made to bring the multitudinous theories into line, to find some fundamental

---

[14] Die *Psychische Krankenbehandlung in ihren Wissenschaftlichen Grundlagen.* By Berthold Kern. Berlin, 1910.

proposition or hypothesis which could be applied universally. Naturally we could not, expect that the layman would discover the missing clue in the review and the leading article referred to above, for both notices were couched in scientific and cautious terms, and the use of headlines in the daily press has so affected the general sense of proportion that the most startling statement passes unnoticed unless sufficiently heralded and advertised by devices of type and superlative redundancies of language. But before I proceed to any statement of these views of Professor Kern, which, are so startlingly in accord with those I have set forth above,[15] I will examine briefly one or two of the opinions given by those eminent medical men whose names I have given.

Sir Clifford Allbutt, who admits to being 'painfully aware' that his reflections are 'tentative and inconclusive,' falls back on the old *a priori* religious grounds, and founds his main argument on the influences of 'Solace Reanimation, and Readjustment.' He is plainly conscious of the general inapplicability of his theory, and the following quotation illustrates forcibly enough how he has been forced to reject the possibilities of a wider hypothesis by his adherence to a narrowing conception. Thus, in speaking of religious forces he says:—

'On the spiritual side the unquestionably genuine phenomena of Conversion point to such changes, to new tides so swift and voluminous as to swing the system out of previous equipoises, and to move to some large measure. And if unhappily the new equilibrium be too often transitory, if too often the *bondage of older habits* drags the system down again to its former and lower mean position, yet in many instances the new position is maintained permanently.'

Here the inherent weakness lies in the phrase which I have put in italics. The reader who has followed my argument through this little work will see at once that Sir Clifford Allbutt's method of cure by faith or conversion does not generally affect the objective mind in its relation to the bodily functions. The change of habit is not permanent in the majority of cases, and even in the remnant where a new outlook persists, it is but a change from one habit to

---

[15] Also my pamphlet 'Re-education of Kinæsthetic Systems.' London, 1908, now reprinted in this volume.

another, the new habit being no more under objective, conscious control than the old one.

Sir Henry Morris finds a common base of 'suggestion' common to all theories of mesmerism, hypnotism, animal magnetism, mental-healing, faith-healing, and Christian Science, and he defines 'suggestion' as the 'enforcing influence of an idea,' but he is analytic rather than synthetic. I agree with much that he writes, especially with regard to what he terms 'The Creative Lie,' the ungrounded statement or suggestion which becomes the basis of a fashion, a scare, or a creed, as the case may be; but the whole article, though scholarly, is chiefly destructive and not materially helpful, and under it all lies, apparently, that conception of a 'sub-conscious self,' which I have tried to controvert in my third chapter.

Dr. H. T. Butlin, while he is prepared. to admit that *'a case of true organic disease may be cured'* (my own italics), seems to look always to faith as the agent, and for this reason I shall not discuss his article here, since it will fall under the general examination of what must be understood by this vague term 'faith' and the same criticism applies also to the contribution of Dr. William Osler.

A summary of these and other articles by prominent medical men may be found in the following quotation from one of our leading morning journals: 'The general trend of scientific and medical thought just now leads more and more away from material theories, and whereas a few years ago the medical profession as a whole firmly refused to consider any form of treatment of which the essential factors could not be either handled in the form of apparatus or weighed in the balance as drugs, we now find the pendulum of medical thought swinging back to conceptions of mental and spiritual healing.' I cannot but express my admiration for the direction in which the swing of the pendulum is setting, at the same time expressing also my regret that it is being held back by all the old encumbrances and rigidities of academic preconception and scientific methods. We can see plainly enough from this symposium of opinion that almost against its will, the medical profession has been forced to admit that cures which in more ignorant times would have been called miraculous, have been effected by mental agencies, that even organic diseases such as cancer have been eliminated without operations or the use of drugs. But still, desperately as it were, there is a clinging to some older form of explanation. Faith, suggestion, the conception of a sub-conscious self which is another form of the soul or spirit, are put forward to account for those things which seem unaccountable on the purely material hypothesis; but I have not found any theory in the articles I have so far instanced which puts forward any explanation of the phenomena that might reasonably be supposed to account for these various origins; not one of these eminent article writers has been able to lay a finger upon any common factor.

Nevertheless, we are confronted with one word which is dominant, and by its iteration must produce an effect on the mind of all readers, whether of this issue of the *British Medical Journal*, or of the various notices which have since appeared in the daily press. That word is 'faith,' and because it is so prominent and so little understood, I feel that it is essential I should give some explanation of it in the light of my own principles.

In the first place, it is, perhaps, hardly necessary for me to point out that faith in this connection need not be allied with any conception of creed or religion. It is true that this is the form in which we are most familiar with it in mental-healing, and the associations which are grouped round the word itself very commonly induce us to connect it with the conceptions that have had such a wide and general influence on the thoughts of mankind in all stages of civilization. But we have abundant evidence now before us that in healing it is the attitude of mind that is of the first importance, and that faith is every whit as effective when directed towards the person of the healer, a drug, or the medicinal qualities supposed to be possessed by a glass of pure water, as when it is directed to a belief in some supernal agency. This fact is indisputable, and it is only because the latter form of faith is so much more widespread, inasmuch as the very essence of all religions necessitates an exercise of this quality, that this agency has effected a number of cures out of all proportion to those brought about by faith in some purely material object. What I here intend by faith, therefore, is its exercise in the widest sense and without any restriction of creed.

So far as we can analyse the effect of what we call an act of faith on the mental processes, it would seem that it is operative in two directions. The first is purely emotional. The patient having conceived a whole-hearted belief that he is going to be delivered from his pain or disease by means of agency supernal or material, experiences a sensation of profound, relief and joy. He understands and believes that without effort on his own part he is to be cured by an apparent miracle, and the effect upon him is to produce a strong, if evanescent, emotional happiness. In this we have an exact parallelism between the patient whose cure is physical and material, and the convert whose cure is spiritual. Now it is widely acknowledged by scientists and the medical profession generally that this condition of happiness is an ideal condition for the sufferer, that it is not only the most hopeful condition of mind, but that it actually produces chemical changes in the physical constitution, which changes are those most salutary in producing a vital condition of the blood, and hence of the organisms.

The second direction in which this act of faith operates is to break down a whole set of mental habits, and substitute for them a new set. The new habits, may or may not be beneficial from the outset apart from the effect produced by the emotional state—which is hardly ever maintained for a long period—but even so the breaking down of the old habits of thought does produce such an effect as will in some cases influence the whole arrangement of the cells forming the tissues and dissipate a morbid condition such as cancer.

Thus we see that this so-called act of faith is in reality purely material in its action, and there is no reason why we should have recourse to it to produce the same and greater effects. It may, perhaps, be asked by some objectors why we should seek to dismiss the act of faith since it undoubtedly produces these ideal conditions in some cases. The answer is obvious. Faith-healing is dangerous in its practice and uncertain it its results. It is dangerous, because in a majority of cases its professors seek in the first place to alleviate pain, which may be done, leaving the disease itself untouched, and, as I have already pointed out in this brochure, in such cases the disease will continue and eventually kill the patient, even though he may be able successfully to fight the pain. Faith-healing is uncertain in its results, because in addition to the danger I have mentioned, it merely substitutes one uncontrolled habit of thought for another. At first the new habit, because it is new, may bring about a change to a better condition, but if it remains it will, in its turn, become stereotyped, and may just as well lead at last to a morbid condition as the old mental habit is superseded. For these reasons, which are trenchant enough, I think, I desire most earnestly to see all the present conceptions that surround this profession of faith-healing thrown aside in order that we may arrive at a sane and reasoned process of mental therapeutics. Let us now turn for a moment to the pronouncements of Professor Kern.[16] Omitting the philosophical aspects of his theory, I will begin by quoting a passage from the third column of the review on page 1499 of the number I have referred to, as follows:—

'...dismissing any naïve interaction theory, he (Professor Kern) firmly maintains there is a continual transformation of mental into bodily processes in action during our whole life. "Mental processes, after they have become developed, accustomed, and habitual, become automatic, and finally purely bodily and mechanical."'

On this point, I think I have already insisted sufficiently, and need only break my quotation in order to emphasize the similarity of thought between the Opinions of Professor Kern, and those I had expressed before reading this notice. We come now to the question of treatment which the writer expounds thus:—

'Turning to the application of his theory to mental therapeutics, Professor Kern discusses the means or methods of psychotherapy, the nature of their action, and the indications and conditions for their employment. First with regard to therapeutic measures, and accepting the fact that psychotherapy has as its point of application the ideal life, Professor Kern stands firmly on the ground that a sharp distinction between psychic and somatic therapy is impossible, seeing that the bodily and mental series are at bottom identical, and that psychic therapy must, therefore, depend on the employment of physical means of some order or another. The sole difference between psycho-therapy and somato-therapy lies in the fact that the former aims at engaging and influencing the consciousness of the subject, whereas the latter does not. Under therapeutic means, therefore, Professor Kern includes all stimuli...which are capable of setting in activity some, or inhibiting other, neuro-cerebral tracts which, either by racial or individual use, have acquired certain associations and memorial or emotional values,

---

[16] Unfortunately I have not been able to obtain any English translation of the work cited above, and must therefore depend on the very able expositions of the leader-writer and the reviewer published in the *British Medical Journal* for June, 1910.

and which, being regarded subjectively, are conscious or mental in character. It will be observed that use, which is also the essence of recollection, furnishes Professor Kern not only guidance as to the means of psychotherapy, but also the fundamental explanation of its action; that is, it is by the employment of definite and carefully chosen physical stimuli which excite neuro-cerebral complexes possessing marked conscious and particularly emotional values of service to the individual, that psychotherapy must act.'

This is, with minor exceptions, merely a scientific statement of the theory I have put forth, and I need only confirm the likeness by one more note from Professor Kern's book, this time a translation of a short passage provided by the writer of the leading article in the *British Medical Journal*:—

'We have here not merely co-ordination, not merely parallelism, but transformation. The supposed antithesis, the difference in kind between mental and bodily processes, vanishes under our hands, and their identical nature presses upon us irresistibly if we are sufficiently unprejudiced and not self-deceived by false conceptions, such as "unconscious thought" and the like.'

Professor Kern's theory is thus seen to be the same in all essentials as that which I have held for many years, upon which I have based the principles of my practice, and which I have thus put to the one and only test. My experience during seventeen years has been by no means a small one, and perhaps no better proof could be afforded of the successful working of the theory when applied to the facts of physical life, than the issue of this brochure and my own very earnest desire that the principles and details of my methods should in the near future be made more widely known.

For it is essential that the peoples of civilization should comprehend the value of their inheritance, that outcome of the long process of evolution which will enable them to govern the uses of their own physical mechanisms. By and through consciousness and the application of a reasoning intelligence, man may rise above the powers of all disease and physical disabilities. This triumph is not to be won in sleep, in trance, in submission, in paralysis, or in anæsthesia, but in a clear, open-eyed, reasoning, deliberate consciousness and apprehension of the wonderful potentialities possessed by mankind, the transcendent inheritance of a conscious mind.

THE THEORY AND PRACTICE
OF A NEW METHOD OF RESPIRATORY
RE-EDUCATION

'Whoever hesitates to utter that which he thinks the highest truth, lest it should be too much in advance of the time, may reassure himself by looking at his acts from an impersonal point of view. ... It is not for nothing that he has in him these sympathies with some principles and repugnance to others. He, with all his capacities, and aspirations, and beliefs, is not an accident, but a product of the time. He must remember that while he is a descendant of the past he is a parent of the future; and that his thoughts are as children born to him, which he may not carelessly let die.' — HERBERT SPENCER

INTRODUCTORY

I T may be of interest to my readers to know that the method I have founded is the result of a practical and unique experience, for my knowledge was gained—

1. While vainly attempting to eradicate personal, vocal, and respiratory defects by recognized systems.

2. While afterwards putting into practice certain original principles, which enabled me to eradicate these defects.

3. While giving personal demonstrations of the application of these principles from a respiratory, vocal, and health-giving point of view.

I first imparted the method thus evolved to patients recommended by medical men over ten years prior to June 1904. At that date I introduced it to leading London medical men, who, after investigation, decided that the method was, as one doctor put it, 'the most efficient known to [him].'

The method makes for—

In *Education*:

1. Prevention of certain defects herein after referred to.

2. Adequate and correct use of the muscular mechanisms concerned with respiration.

In *Re-education*:

1. Eradication of certain defects hereinafter referred to.

2. Co-ordination in the use of the muscular mechanisms concerned with respiration.

The result of (2) is not only to make that function efficient, but also to insure that normal activity and natural massage of the *internal organs* so necessary to the adequate performance of the vital functions and the preservation of a proper condition of health.

F. MATTHIAS ALEXANDER

22 ARMY AND NAVY MANSIONS,
VICTORIA STREET, LONDON, S.W.,
January, 1907.

I.
THE THEORY OF RESPIRATORY RE-EDUCATION

THE artificial conditions of modern civilized life, among which is comparative lack of free exercise in the open air, are conducive to the *in*adequate use of breathing power. Indulgence in harmful habits of feeding and posture have caused these same habits, by heredity and unconscious imitation, to become 'second nature' in the great majority of adults to-day, and frequently in children, even at an early age.

The normal condition of vigor in the action of the component parts of the respiratory mechanisms is greatly interfered with; general nervous relaxation is brought about, and a feeble, flabby action becomes permanent.

Some muscles of the thoracic mechanism are used solely for regular performance of the breathing movements which were never intended by Nature to monopolize the particular act, but only to serve as a relief or change, while those which should take the lead remain entirely inert for the greater part of life; hence arises a condition in which the posture, the symmetry of the body, the graceful normal curves of the whole frame, suffer alteration and change.

The capacity and mobility of the thorax (chest) are decreased, its shape (particularly in the lumbar region, clavicles, and lower sides of the chest) is changed in a harmful way, and the abdominal viscera displaced; while the heart, lungs and other vital organs are allowed to drop below their normal position. Inadequate holding-space of the thorax—which means a distinct lessening of the 'vital capacity'—and displacement of the vital organs within it, are great factors in retarding the natural activity of the parts concerned, and are thereby responsible for their inability fully and naturally to perform their functions. The natural chemical changes in the human organism cannot, under these circumstances, be adequate.

The serious interference with the circulatory processes, and the inadequate oxygenation of the blood, mean that the system will not be properly nourished and cleansed of impurities, for the action of the excretory processes will be impeded, and the whole organism slowly but surely charged with foreign matter, which, sooner or later, causes acute symptoms of disease.

It will at once be understood that the defects enumerated produce distinct deterioration in the condition of the different organs of the body, and it is well known that an organ's power of resistance to disease depends upon the adequacy of its functioning power, which in turn depends upon adequate activity.

Records exist which prove that the Chinese physicians employed breathing exercises in the treatment of certain diseases 2000 B.C. It is therefore obvious that the people concerned had reached—

1. A stage in their evolution which corresponds with that of our time—*i.e.*, demanding re-education.

2. A stage of observation of cause and effect similar to that of to-day, which led them to see the need of re-education, such re-education being essential to the restoration of the natural conditions present at birth in every normal babe, though gradually deteriorated under conditions of modern life.

In recent years the following members of the medical profession have urged the inestimable value of the cultivation and development of the respiratory mechanism, and their conclusions have been borne out by the practical results secured by respiratory re-education combined with proper medical treatment.

MEDICAL OPINIONS CONCERNING THE EVIL EFFECT OF INTERFERENCE WITH AND INADEQUATE USE OF THE RESPIRATORY PROCESSES

Dr. Scanes Spicer, Surgeon, Diseases of the Throat, St. Mary's Hospital, in a debate on the value of 'Respiratory Exercises, etc.,' published in the *British Medical Journal*, vol. ii., 1902, p. 690, said: 'As a matter of fact, the manner of breathing of every child, just as much as its food and clothing, housing and air, exercise, bathing, and education, require constant and unremitting attention from the moment of birth.'

Mr. W. Arbuthnot Lane, surgeon to Guy's Hospital, in his lecture published in the *Lancet*, December 17, 1904, p. 1697, urges that reduction in the respiratory capacity is a very great factor in lowering the activity of all the vital processes of the body, and that in the first instance inadequate aeration and oxygenation is the result of serious alteration in the abdominal mechanisms, and afterwards the insufficient aeration impairs the digestive processes.

Dr. Hugh A. McCallum, in his clinical lecture on 'Visceroptosis' (dropping of the viscera), as published in the *British Medical Journal*, February 18, 1905, p.345, points out that over ninety percent of the females suffering from neurasthenia (exhaustion of nerve force) are victims of visceroptosis, and that the conditions present are bad standing posture, imperfect use of the lower zone of the thorax, and the lack of tone in the abdominal muscular system which leads to defective intra-abdominal pressure. He also mentions that Dr. John Madison Taylor of Philadelphia and Keith of England were the two first to point out that the origin of this disease begins in a faulty position and use of the thorax.

In a leading article in the *Lancet*, December 24, 1904, p. 1796: 'Whatever may be the causes, it is certain that an increasing number of town-dwellers suffer from constipation and atony of the colon, and that purgatives, enemata, and massage are powerless to prevent their progress from constipation to coprostasis.'

CONVALESCENTS

The value of respiratory re-education in the treatment of convalescents was pointed out recently (1905) by M. Siredey and M. Rosenthal in a paper read at a meeting of the Société Médicale des Hopitaux.

Excerpt from the *Lancet*, February 18, 1905, p. 463:

'They said that respiratory insufficiency was one of the causes of the general debility which showed itself after an acute illness. It was easily recognized by the following symptoms, which the patient presented— namely, thoracic insufficiency, shown by absence or impairment of the movements of the thorax; and diaphragmatic insufficiency, shown by immobility or recession of the abdomen during inspiration—a condition met with in pseudo-pleurisy of the bases of the lungs.

'Respiratory re-education was, in their opinion, the specific treatment for respiratory insufficiency. In the case of convalescents it constantly produced a progressive three-fold effect—namely, expansion of the thorax, diuresis, and increase of weight. It promoted in a marked degree the recuperation of the vital functions which followed acute illness, and the general health of the patients improved rapidly. It ought to be combined with other forms of treatment, and the action of the latter was enhanced by it.'

The matter of preventing defective and restoring proper action clearly calls for attention. The foregoing will enable the reader definitely to understand what is necessary—viz.:

1. *In Prevention.*—The inculcation of a proper mental attitude towards the act of breathing in children, to be followed by those detailed instructions necessary to the correct practice of such respiratory exercises as will maintain adequate and proper use of the breathing organs.

2. *In Restoration.*—A body possessing one or other or all of the defects previously named will need re-education in order to eradicate the defects brought about by bad habits, etc., and restore a proper condition. As the breathing mechanism is ordinarily *unconsciously* controlled, it is necessary, in order to regain full, efficiency in the use of it, to proceed by way of *conscious* control until the normal conditions return. Afterwards, when perfected, unconscious control—as it originally existed prior to respiratory and physical deterioration—will supervene.

II.
ERRORS TO BE AVOIDED AND FACTS TO BE REMEMBERED IN THE THEORY AND PRACTICE OF RESPIRATORY RE-EDUCATION

'Each faculty acquires fitness for its function by performing its function; and if its function is performed for it by a substituted agency, none of the required adjustment of nature takes place; but the nature becomes deformed to fit the artificial arrangements instead of the natural arrangements.' — HERBERT SPENCER

ANYTHING that makes for good may be rendered harmful in its effect by injudicious application or improper use, and many authorities have referred to this fact in connection with breathing exercises. For the guidance of my readers I will detail some of the harmful results which accrue from the attempt to take what are known as 'deep breaths' during the practice of breathing and physical exercises, in accordance with instructions set down and principle advocated in recognized breathing systems.

At the outset, let me point out that respiratory education, or respiratory re-education will not prove successful unless the mind of the pupil is thoroughly imbued with the true principles which apply to atmospheric pressure, the equilibrium of the body, the centre of gravity, and to positions of mechanical advantage where the alternate expansions and contractions of the thorax are concerned. In other words, *it is essential to have a proper mental attitude towards respiratory education or re-education, and the specific acts which constitute the exercises embodied* in it, together with a proper knowledge and practical employment of the *true primary movement* in each and every act. I may remark that I recognized this factor and put it to practical use over twelve years ago, but it has been quite overlooked or neglected in the other systems formulated before and since that time. In fact, when I introduced my method to leading London medical men they quickly admitted the value of this

64

important factor, and expressed their surprise that it had not been previously advocated as such, seeing that from a practical point of view it is so essential, not only in the eradication of respiratory faults or defects (re-education) but also in preventing them (education).

A proper mental attitude, let me repeat, then, is all-important. From the absence of it arise many of the serious defects ordinarily met with in the respiratory mechanism of civilized people, all of which are exaggerated in the practice of customary 'breathing exercises.'

1. *'Sniffing'* or *'Gasping'*—If the 'deep breath' be taken through the nasal passages there will be a loud 'sniffing' sound and collapse of the alæ nasi, and if through the mouth, a 'gasping' sound. The pupil has not been told that if the thorax is expanded correctly the lungs will at once be filled with air by atmospheric pressure, exactly as a pair of bellows is filled when the handles are pulled apart.

It is a well-known fact, but one greatly to be regretted, that all who have taken lessons in London from teachers of breathing and physical exercises actually are told that, in order to get the increased air-supply, they *must* 'sniff.'

But, worse than this, many medical men are guilty of similar instruction to their patients; and when giving a personal demonstration of how a 'deep breath' should be taken, they 'sniff' loudly and bring about a collapse of the alæ nasi, throw back the head, and interfere with the centre of gravity. Of course, it is only necessary to remind them of the law of atmospheric pressure as it applies to breathing, and they at once recognize their error.

Such a state of affairs serves to show that lamentable ignorance prevails even in the twentieth century in connection with so essential a function as breathing; and reflection causes one to realize the seriousness of a situation which, from some points of view, is really pathetic.

Most people, if asked to take a 'deep breath,' will proceed to—I use the phrase spoken by thousands of people I have experimented upon—'suck air into the lungs to expand the chest,' whereas, of course, the proper expansion of the chest, as a primary movement, causes the alæ nasi to be dilated and the lungs to be instantly filled with air by atmospheric pressure, without any harmful lowering of the pressure.

2. During this harmful 'sniffing' act it will be seen that—

(*a*) The larynx is unduly depressed; likewise the diaphragm.

The undue strain, caused by this unnatural crowding down of the larynx and its accessories, is undoubtedly the greatest factor in the causation of throat troubles, especially when professional voice-users are concerned as the practical tests I have made during the past twelve years have abundantly proved. My success in London with eminent members of the dramatic and vocal profession, sent to me by their medical advisers, might be mentioned in this connection.

(*b*) The upper chest is unduly raised, and in most cases the shoulders also.

(*c*) The back is unduly hollowed in the lumbar region.

(*d*) The abdomen is generally protruded, and there is abnormally deranged intra-abdominal pressure.

(*e*) The head is thrown too far back, and the neck duly tensed and shortened at a time when it should be perfectly free from strain.

(*f*) Parts of the chest are unduly expanded, while others that should share in the expansion are contracted, particularly the back in the lumbar region.

(*g*) During the expiration there is an undue falling of the upper chest, which harmfully increases the intrathoracic pressure, and so dams back the blood in the thin-walled veins and auricles and hampers the heart's action.

(*h*) Undue larynx depression prevents the proper placing and natural movements of the tongue, the adequate and correct opening of the mouth for the formation of the resonance cavity necessary to the vocalization of a true 'Ah.'

It is well known that the tongue is attached to the larynx, and therefore any undue depression of the latter must of necessity interfere with the free and correct movements of the former.

(*i*) The head is thrown back to open the mouth.

This is a common fault, even with professional singers, and a moment's consideration of the movements of the jaw—from an anatomical point of view—will show that it should move downwards without effort, and that it is not necessary to move the head back wards in order to effect the opening of the mouth by the lowering of the jaw, since, as a matter of fact, the latter movement will be more readily and perfectly performed if the head remains erect without any deviatory posture.

Every voice-user should learn to open the mouth without throwing back the head. Very distinct benefits will accrue to those who succeed in establishing this habit.

It is well known that the practice of 'physical-culture' exercises has caused emphysema, and it has been suggested that unnatural breathing exercises have also been responsible for the condition. I refer to this because I wish to show that it would not be possible to cause emphysema by the method of respiratory education and re-education I have formulated.

Emphysema may be caused by—

1. The reduction of the elasticity of the lung cells and tissue resulting from undue expansion of the lungs and their being held too long in this expanded position.

2. The undue intrathoracic pressure—during an attempt at expiration or some physical act—upon the air cells, which remain filled with air in consequence of the means of egress from the lungs being temporarily closed by the approximation of vocal reeds and ventricular bands.

If the fundamental principles of my method are observed, these conditions cannot be present during the practice of the exercises, and, therefore, emphysema not only cannot be produced, but even is likely to be remedied when previously existing.

In the first place, the tendency unduly to expand any part or parts of the thorax in particular, to the exclusion of other parts, is prevented by the detailed personal instruction given in connection with each exercise in its application to individual defects or peculiarities of the pupil. Moreover, the mechanical advantages in the body-pose and chest-poise assumed in these exercises cause them to be performed with the minimum of effort, and lead to an even and controlled expansion of the whole thorax. There is not, as is too often the case an undue expansion of one part of the chest, while other parts, which should share in such expansion, are being contracted—a condition that obtains, for instance, when the diaphragm is unduly depressed in inspiration.

There is, then, a sinking above and below the clavicles, a hollowing in the lumbar region of the back, undue protrusion of the abdomen, displacement of the abdominal viscera, reduction in height, undue depression of the larynx, and the centre of gravity is thrown too far back.

The *striking feature* in those who have *practised customary breathing exercises* is an *undue lateral expansion* of the lower ribs, when several or all of the above defects are present. This excessive expansion gives an undue width to the lower part of the chest, and there are thousands of young girls who present quite a matronly appearance in consequence. The breathing exercises imparted by teachers of singing are particularly effective in bringing about this undesirable and harmful condition.

> The guiding principle that should be invariably kept in mind by both teacher and pupil is to secure, with the minimum of effort, perfect use of the component parts of the mechanisms concerned in respiration and vocalization. Then, sooner or later, adequate mobility, power, speed, absolute control, and artistic manipulation must follow.

Most people—teachers as well as pupils—when thinking of or practising breathing exercises, have one fixed idea—viz, that of causing a *great expansion* of the chest, whereas its proper and adequate *contraction* is equally important. There are, indeed, many cases in which the expiratory movement calls for more attention than the inspiratory.

Careful observation will show that those who take breath by the 'sniffing' or 'gasping' mode of breathing always experience great difficulty with breath-control in speech and song, or during the performance of breathing exercises. This applies equally whether the air is expelled through the mouth or nasal passages, and is due to the imperfect use of the thoracic mechanism, and the consequent loss of mechanical advantage already referred to at the end of the inspiration.

The natural and powerful air-controlling power is, therefore, absent, and its absence causes undue approximation of the vocal reeds, and probably the ventricular bands in the endeavour to prevent the escape of air, which air, when once released under these conditions, is thereafter inadequately and imperfectly controlled.

There is considerable increase in this lack of breath-control in vocal use, the upper chest being more rapidly and forcibly depressed during the vocalization.

It is not a matter of surprise, for, if a mechanical advantage is essential to the proper expansion of the thorax for the intake of air, it is equally essential to the controlling power during the expiration; and if during the expiration the upper chest is falling, it clearly proves that the advantage indicated is not present.

III.
THE PRACTICE OF RESPIRATORY RE-EDUCATION

HABIT IN RELATION TO PECULIARITIES AND DEFECTS

'If we contemplate the method of Nature, we see that everywhere vast results are brought about by accumulating minute actions.'— HERBERT SPENCER

THE mental and physical peculiarities or defects of men and women are the result of heredity or acquired habit, and the most casual observer has noticed that certain peculiarities or defects are characteristic of the members of particular families, as for instance, in connection with the standing and sitting postures, the style of walking, the position of the shoulders and shoulder-blades, the use of the arm, and the use of the vocal organs in speech, etc.

Such family peculiarities or defects are unconsciously acquired by the children, often becoming more pronounced in the second generation; such acquirements making for good or ill, as the case may be. I will, however, confine myself to an enumeration of those with a harmful tendency, as an understanding of bad habits is essential to considering the teaching principles adopted in my method of respiratory-physical re-education.

The chief peculiarities or defects may be broadly indicated as—

1. An incorrect mental attitude towards the respiratory act.
2. Lack of control over, and improper and inadequate use of, the component parts of the different mechanisms of the body, limbs, and nervous system.
3. Incorrect pose of the body and chest poise, and therefrom consequent defects in the standing and sitting postures; the interference with the normal position and shape of the spine, as well as the ribs, the costal arch, the vital organs and the abdominal viscera.

Re-education, when one or other or all of these peculiarities or defects are present, means eradication of existing bad habits, and the following will indicate some of the chief principles upon which the teaching method of this re-education is based:—

That where the human machinery is concerned Nature does not work in parts, but treats everything as a whole.

That a proper mental attitude towards respiration is at once inculcated, and each and every respiratory act in the practice of the exercises is the direct result of volition; the primary, secondary and other movements necessary to the proper performance of such act having first been definitely indicated to the pupil.

It may prove of interest to mention that W. Marcet, M.D., F.R.S. and Harry Campbell, M.D., B.S., London, are of opinion that volition as such makes a direct demand upon the breathing powers, quite apart from all physical effort, and with these great advantages, that, unlike the latter, it neither increases the production of waste products nor tends to cause thoracic rigidity, thus more or less retarding the movements of the chest. The experiments made by Dr. Marcet show that the duration of a man's power to sustain the muscle contraction necessary to raise a weight a given number of times depends upon the endurance of the brain-centres causing the act of violation rather than upon the muscular power. An instance is quoted of a man who lifted a weight of 4 pounds 203 times, and who, after resting and performing forced breathing movements, raised the same weight to the same height 700 times.

Regarding muscle development and chest expansion, Dr. Harry Campbell has in his book on breathing taken the case of Sandow. His conclusion will prove of interest. He pointed out that Sandow claimed to be able to increase the size of the chest 14 inches—that is, from 48 to 62 inches in circumference. Dr. Campbell then expressed the opinion that this increase is almost entirely the result of the swelling up of the large muscles surrounding the chest, and that most probably the increase in his bony chest (thorax) is not more than 2 to 3 inches, seeing that his 'vital capacity' is only 275 cubic inches.

(For ten years past I have drawn the attention of medical men to the deception of ordinary chest measurements and to the evils wrought by the physical training and the 'stand-at-attention' attitude in vogue in the army, and also to the harmful effects of the drill in our schools, where the unfortunate children are made to assume a posture which is exactly that of the

71

soldier, whose striking characteristic is the undue and harmful hollow in the lumbar spine and the numerous defects that are inseparable from this unnatural posture.)

There is such immediate improvement in the pose of the body and poise of the chest (whatever the conditions, excepting, of course, organized structural defects) that a valuable mechanical advantage is secured in the respiratory movements, and this is gradually improved by the practice until the habit becomes established, and the law of gravity appertaining to the human body is duly obeyed.

The mechanical advantage referred to is of particular value, for it means prevention of undue and harmful falling of the upper chest at the end of the expiration, which is always present in those who practise the customary breathing exercises, the pupil being then deprived of the mechanical advantage so essential to the proper performance of the next inspiratory act.

Then follows due increase in the movements of expansion and contraction of the thorax until such movements are adequate and perfectly controlled.

Further, these expansions are primary movements in securing that increase in the capacity of the chest necessary to afford the normal oscillations of atmospheric pressure, without unduly lowering that pressure—opportunity to fill the lungs with air, while the contractions overcome the air pressure and force the air out of the lungs, and at the same time constitute the controlling power of the speed and length of the expiration.

The excessive and harmful lowering of the air pressure in the respiratory tract, and the consequent collapse of the alæ nasi, is prevented by so regulating the respiratory speed that the lungs are filled by atmospheric pressure.

The value of this will be readily understood when it is remembered that such lowering, which is always present in the 'sniffing' mode of breathing, causes collapse of the alæ nasi. It also tends to cause congestion of the mucous membrane of the respiratory tract on the sucker system, setting up catarrh and its attendant evils, such as throat disorders, loss of voice, bronchitis, asthma, and other pulmonary troubles.

From the first lesson the effect upon the splanchnic area is such that the blood is more or less drawn away from it to the lungs, and is then evenly distributed to other parts of the body. The intra-abdominal pressure is more or less raised, and there is a gradual tendency to the permanent establishment of normal conditions.

The use of bandages or corsets is to be condemned as treatment in protruding abdomen instead of adopting practical means to remove the cause. Such support to the abdominal wall is artificial and harmful, since it tends to make the muscles more flaccid. The respiratory mechanism should be re-educated, for this would mean a re-education or strengthening of the supports Nature has supplied. In other words, the sinking above and below the clavicles and the undue hollowing of the lumbar spine—the great factors in the direct causation of the protrusion of the abdomen—are removed, and a normal condition of the abdominal muscles established. This means a very decided improvement in the figure and general health.

The improvement in the abdominal conditions (the improved position of the abdominal visceral and the development of the abdominal muscles) is proportionate to that of the respiratory movements—a fact that can be readily understood when I point out that the movements of the parts are interdependent. When the faulty distension of the splanchnic area is present it will be found that the diaphragm is unduly low in breathing; and when there is excessive depression of the diaphragm in respiration there is interference with the centre of gravity by displacement forward, and the compensatory arching back ward in the lumbar region.

After a time there is such improvement in the use of the component parts of the mechanism that an inspiration may, if desired, be secured by a depression of the diaphragm, while at the same moment the condition in the splanchnic area is actually improved.

Improvement in respiratory exchange is secured by gradual increase in the expansions and contractions of the thorax, which increase the aeration of lungs, the supply of oxygen, and the elimination of CO_2.

The quantity of residual air in the lungs is greatly increased, and by always converting the expired air into a controlled whispered vowel during the practice of the breathing exercises very great benefits accrue—notably those derived from the prolonged interthoracic pressure necessary to force the adequate supply of oxygen into the blood and eliminate the due quantity of CO_2.

Employment of these whispered tones means the proper use of the vocal organs in a form of vocalization little associated with ordinary bad habits, and that perfect co-ordination of the parts concerned which is inseparable from adequately controlled whisper vocalization.

There is a rapid clearing of the skin, the white face becoming a natural colour, and a reduction of fat in the obese by its being burnt off with the extra oxygen supply.

This reduction in the weight and size is often quite remarkable, as also the development of the flaccid muscles of the abdominal wall and the consequent improvement in the activity of the parts concerned.

CONCLUDING REMARKS

THE foregoing will serve to draw attention to the far-reaching and beneficial effects of what, for the lack of a more satisfactory and comprehensive name, I refer to as respiratory re-education.

It is a method that makes for the maintenance and restoration of those physical conditions possessed by every normal child at birth, the presence of which insures a proper standard of health, adequate resistance to disease, and a reserve power which, if a serious illness should occur, will serve to turn the tide at the critical moment towards recovery. The insurance of such a condition for a generation would mean the regeneration of the human race as constituted to-day; and I have no hesitation in stating that the results secured during the past twelve years, and particularly during the past two and a half years in London in co-operation with leading medical men, justify me in asserting that the practical application of the principles of this new method in education and re-education will be invaluable in overcoming the disadvantages and bad habits of our artificial civilized life, and prove the great factor in successfully checking the physical degeneration of mankind.

RE-EDUCATION OF THE KINÆSTHETIC SYSTEMS CONCERNED WITH THE DEVELOPMENT OF ROBUST PHYSICAL WELL-BEING

EDUCATION

'It is because the body is a machine that education is possible. Education is the formation of habits, a superinducing of an artificial organization upon the natural organization of the body; so that acts, which at first require a conscious effort, eventually become unconscious and mechanical.' — HUXLEY

RE-EDUCATION

'It is because the body is a machine that (RE)education is possible. (RE)education is the formation of (NEW AND CORRECT) habits, a (RE-INSTATING OF THE CORRECT) artificial organization upon the natural organization of the body; so that acts, which at first require conscious effort eventually become unconscious and mechanical.'

22 ARMY AND NAVY MANSIONS,
VICTORIA STREET, LONDON, S.W.
December, 1908.

THE DOCTRINES OF ANTAGONISTIC ACTION AND MECHANICAL ADVANTAGE

In the process of *creating* a co-ordination one psycho-physical factor provides a position of rigidity by means of which the moving parts are held to the mode in which their function is carried on.

This psycho-physical factor also constitutes a steady and firm condition which enables the Directive Agent of the sphere of consciousness to discriminate the action of the kinæsthetic and motion agents which it must maintain without any interference or discontinuity.

The whole condition which thus obtains is herein termed 'antagonistic action,' and the attitude of rigidity essential as a factor in the process is called the position of 'mechanical advantage.'

A PRESENTATION OF PRINCIPLES AND LAWS

Exemplified in Mr. F. Matthias Alexander's Method of the

RE-EDUCATION OF THE KINAESTHETIC SYSTEMS

(SENSORY APPRECIATION OF MUSCULAR MOVEMENT)

Concerned with the Development of Robust Physical Well-being.

B
Y this process of Re-education an effective installation is made of the reflex muscular systems involved through the creation of an intelligent directive power on the part of the individual, thus removing a crude and useless *kinaesthesis*, which must be regarded as either debauched or deformed, and establishing one of valid and unfailing function.

By the preliminary, and temporary, employment of a group of exercises of ideo-motor nature an induction is gradually assured of an automatic sensori-motor activity, by which correct and healthy bodily movements and poses are always certain without further attention on the part of the individual, except such as a very brief daily exercise may demand.

In explanation of the object, thus defined and of the mode in which that object is to be attained, the notice of the student is directed to the following postulates:—

1. That when defects in the poise of the body, in the pose of the chest, in the use of the muscular mechanisms, and in the equilibrium are present in the human being the condition thus evidenced is an *undue rigidity* of parts of the muscular mechanisms associated with *undue flaccidity* of others. This undue rigidity is always found in those parts of the muscular mechanisms which are forced to perform duties other than those intended by nature, and are consequently ill-adapted for their function.

Herbert Spencer writes:—

'Each faculty acquires fitness for its function by performing its function; and if its function is performed for it by a substituted agency none of the required adjustment of nature takes place; but the nature becomes deformed to fit the artificial arrangements instead of the natural arrangements.'

2. That it is essential at the outset of re-education to bring about the relaxation of the unduly rigid parts of the muscular mechanisms in order to secure the correct use of the inadequately employed and wrongly coordinated parts.

In a previous publication, 'Why Deep Breathing and Physical Culture Exercises do more harm than good,' I have explained at length that Physical Exercises, as understood in present day 'physical-culture,' actually increase, in the defective subject, that rigidity of which the removal is primarily and vitally important.

3. That all conscious effort exerted in attempts at physical action causes, in the great majority of the people of to-day, such tension of the muscular system concerned as to lead to exaggeration rather than eradication of the defects already present.

I may cite, as examples of such defects, faulty poise of the body and pose of the chest, unstable equilibrium (inability, for instance, to maintain equilibrium during simple movements), undue strain or incorrect use of isolated parts of the muscular system (such as the constant crowding down of the structures of the throat by strain placed upon the larynx and undue depression of that organ), and the performance of functions by one part more properly discharged by another (as when the arms and neck are stiffened in performing acts which properly call for the perfect co-ordination of the muscular mechanisms of the back. The stiffened necks and arms of the people of to-day are outward signs and tokens of the imperfect development and lack of the co-ordination of the muscular system of the back and spine. Such a condition is still being fostered and developed day by day in the children of our schools.)

4. That a directly conscious effort in the performance of the exercise employed in the early stages of re-education (*a*) implies that the pupil relies upon *his own faulty sensations* (that is, he is realizing his sensations) *for*

81

guidance in the correct performance of such exercises—guidance which it is not in the power of the incoherent and often absolutely misleading sensations of the imperfectly coordinated subject to give; and (*b*) produces, as a result of the tension induced by such effort, thoracic rigidity and breathlessness—the one making the correct performance of the exercises impossible, the other interfering with the controlling forces concerned.

5. That it is harmful for teacher and pupil alike if the latter is made to assume, during his exercises, what is usually considered the correct standing position. It is obvious that the same position cannot be correct for every human being, nor even for all who are properly coordinated.

Take the case, for example, of a boy who stoops very much, and combines a sinking above and below the clavicles with abnormal protrusion of the shoulder-blades. If he is told to 'stand up straight' he will at once make undue physical effort to carry out the order thus crudely given, with the result that the shoulders will be thrown backward and upward, the shoulder-blades still further protruded, and the front and upper parts of the chest unduly elevated and expanded. There will also be a narrowing, a sinking, and a flabbiness of the lower dorsal and posterior thoracic region, with corresponding fixed protrusion and rigidity of the front chest wall, undue arching of the lumbar spine, shortening of the boyd and harmful stiffening of the arms and neck; instead of a fullness, broadness and firmness of the back, with free mobility of the chest walls, resulting in normal curve of the lumbar region and comparative lengthening of the spine. With the arms hanging vertically, the relative position of that part of the thorax where the lungs are situated will be seen to be in front of the arms, instead of being, as it should be, behind them. In such a position, the boy feels helpless, and tires rapidly owing to the imperfect co-ordination, and any attempt to accustom him to this erect posture will ultimately result in deterioration rather than improvement.

Now the narrowing and arching of the back already referred to is exactly opposite to what is required by nature, and to that which is obtained in re-education, viz. *widening of the back and a more normal and extended position of the spine.* Moreover, if these conditions of the back be first secured, the neck and arms will no longer be stiffened, and the other faults will be eradicated.

6. That in order to obviate the evils enunciated in the last two postulates the teacher must himself place the pupil in a position of mechanical advantage,

from which the pupil, by the mere mental rehearsal of orders which the teacher will dictate, can *insure the posture specifically correct for himself*, although he is not, as yet, conscious of what that posture is.

I append a simple example of what is meant by mechanical advantage. Let the pupil sit as far back in a chair as possible. The teacher, having decided upon the orders necessary for securing the elongation of spine, the freedom of the neck (*i.e*, requisite natural laxness) and other conditions desirable to the particular case in hand, will then ask the pupil to rehearse them mentally, at the same time that he himself renders assistance by the skilful use of his hands. Then, holding with one hand one or two books, as the case may be, against the inner back of the chair, he will rely upon the pupil inwardly rehearsing the orders necessary to maintain and improve the conditions present, while he, with the other hand placed upon the pupil's shoulder, causes the body gradually to incline backwards until its weight is taken by the back of the chair. The shoulder-blades will, of course, be resting against the books.

7. That the orders to be dictated by the teacher and mentally rehearsed by the pupil are of two kinds:—

(*a*) Concerning definite inhibition.

(*b*) Concerning definite performance.

I may briefly explain (*a*) by stating that the teacher will have to deal with incorrect movements unconsciously performed. These movements, occurring at the moment when he dictates the orders necessary to bring about co-ordination of the different parts of the mechanism, assert themselves and become primary, and hinder the performance of the correct and co-ordinated movements as ordered. It is, therefore, as necessary to order the *inhibition of incorrect and unconsciously performed acts* as to give orders which will secure the co-ordinated use of the mechanisms involved. Therefore, when the teacher has discovered the errors unconsciously committed by the pupil when beginning to rehearse the correct orders, he will draw attention to them, and give a definite order concerning what is *not* to be done, *e.g*., the peculiar bad habit, perhaps, of a lifetime. This negative order must precede all positive commands. In other words, *the order or orders concerning what is not to be done are to be considered as primary, and those concerning what is to be done as secondary.*

8. That in order to secure the results desired, it is essential to teach the pupil to rehearse the dictated orders, not to do exercises, *i.e.*, to devote his attention to *apprehending the instructions of his teacher—those means whereby* he is to gain what he requires, and not, as he will be apt to do, to concentrate his thoughts upon the end sought. The orders are necessarily prior to their execution, and if those dictated by the teacher are correct for the particular case in hand, the mental realization by the pupil will be automatically followed by their correct performance—a co-ordinated association with the ideo-motor impulses.

It is important to remember, however, that in rehearsing the orders dictated by his teacher, the untrained pupil will not merely assent to them, but will believe that he has carried them out as desired. Moreover, though his mental attitude may be correct, and also his rehearsal of the orders, the habit of a lifetime will prove too strong, and he will not be content until he *feels conscious of impressions*, however fallacious these may be, that he has fulfilled the instructions given him. This, of course, means that he is trusting to his own imperfect judgment again, and so reverting to his old bad habits. Now he must not put his own construction upon the instructions given by the teacher—since such construction will be drawn from the *faulty sensations* which he was accustomed to experience in his imperfectly educated state— nor must he, at first, make any endeavour to satisfy himself as to whether the exercise itself has been correctly performed. Until his powers of muscular appreciation infallibly recognize the new correct muscular co-ordinations, he must be guided *solely by his teacher*, and must learn to rehearse the instructions he receives without attempting (as he understands it) to carry them out. With a pupil who is mentally receptive, and who adequately employs his power of inhibition prior to the correct rehearsal of the orders, a skilful teacher may almost perform miracles. For the time being, the pupil places his entire muscular system under the control of his conscious will, directing himself solely according to the suggestion afforded by the orders of the teacher.

Much, has been heard during recent years of physical deterioration, and manifold suggestions have been made as to its causes and the remedies to be adopted. The matter is a simple one.

The Kinæsthetic Systems concerned with correct and healthy bodily movements and postures have become demoralized by the habits engendered in the schoolroom through the restraint enforced at a time when natural activity should have been encouraged and scientifically directed, and in the crouching positions necessitated by useless and irrational deskwork. Muscular and Nervous Systems, the mechanisms of physical existence, have become deteriorated by lack of activity in correct modes, and through failure of the circulatory fluid—vitiated through its inability to secure full co-operation of the all-important respiratory functions—to maintain health-giving metabolic activity.

The method of Re-education of the Kinæsthetic System involved in the development, and the assured continuance of Robust Physical Well-being which is here explained, is offered as an effectual and rational means of removing the effects of those faulty child and adolescent modes of existence to which reference has been made, since it ensures the performance, by each part of the muscular mechanism, of its own specific function, in proper co-ordination with the other parts.

CPSIA information can be obtained
at www.ICGtesting.com
Printed in the USA
LVHW032313280423
745586LV00018B/64